Reflexology

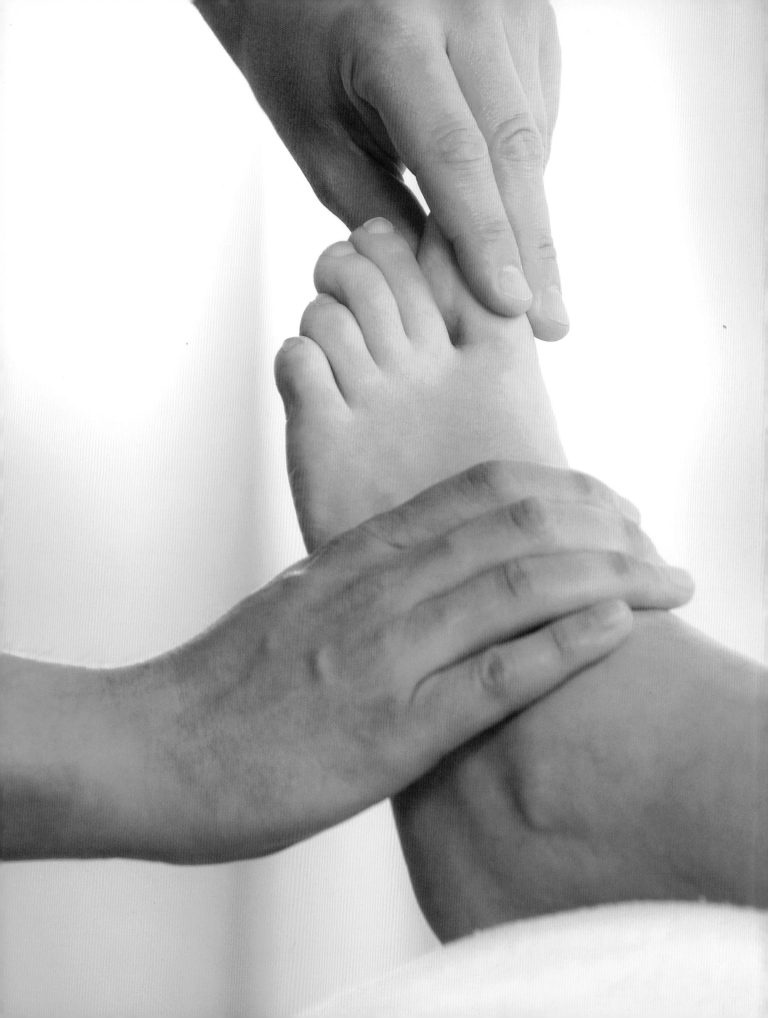

Reflexology

A hands-on approach to your health and well-being

Joëlle Peeters

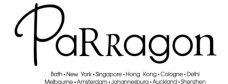

Bath · New York · Singapore · Hong Kong · Cologne · Delhi
Melbourne · Amsterdam · Johannesburg · Auckland · Shenzhen

This edition published by Parragon in 2010

Parragon

Chartist House

15–17 Trim Street

Bath BA1 1HA, UK

www.parragon.com

ISBN: 978-1-4075-1738-4

Printed in China

Produced by the Bridgewater Book Company Ltd

Photography: Simon Punter

contents

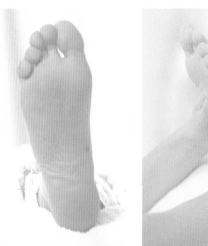

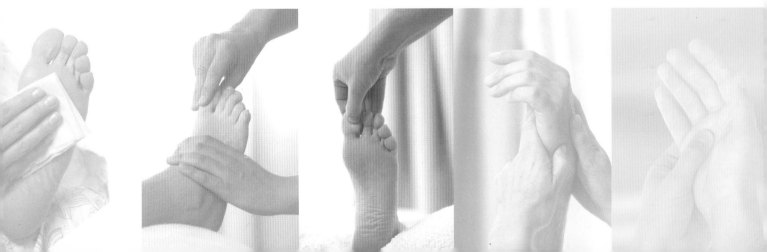

what is reflexology?

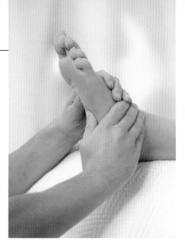

Reflexology functions in two ways: as a diagnostic tool and as a method of treatment. A reflexology treatment can be used for the correction and prevention of ill health.

I t is known that different reflex points found in the feet and hands correspond to an area in the body. By using the thumb and fingers in a particular way to massage the relevant reflex points, pain and other symptoms in the corresponding area of the body can be alleviated. This knowledge probably originated in China, where the Chinese used pressure points on the feet as a form of treatment as long as 5,000 years ago.

The earliest pictorial evidence of reflexology was discovered in the tomb of a physician named Ankm'ahor, at Saqqara in Egypt, dating from around 2,500 to 2,330 BCE. The tomb drawings show practitioners massaging their patients' hands and feet, with the inscription reading "do not hurt me," and "I shall act so you shall praise me."

Evidence has shown that, in more recent times, Native American folk medicine also used a form of foot massage as a healing aid.

In 1917, Dr. William H. Fitzgerald, an ear, nose, and throat consultant in the United States, published the book *Zone Therapy, or Relieving Pain At Home*. He divided the body into ten longitudinal zones (or energy channels)—hence the term "zone therapy."

Dr. Fitzgerald observed that by using, for example, rubber bands or metal combs to apply pressure to fingers or toes, he could bring about an anaesthetizing effect and normalization to all parts of the zone treated.

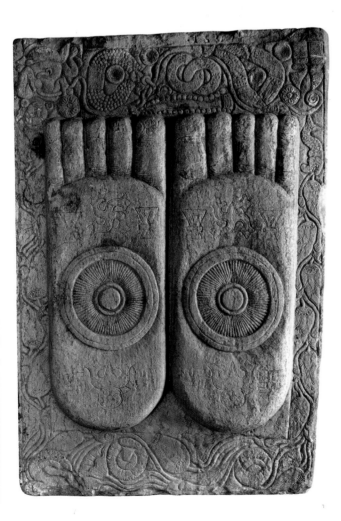

Limestone panel from a first-century BCE Indian sculpture depicting the Buddha's footprints. Feet represent the Buddha's continued presence on Earth, and have long been the focus of respect in India.

Eunice Ingham trained as a remedial therapist, so she had a paramedical background. She is known as "the mother of reflexology" for her work on mapping each reflex and point of contact on the hands and feet to the various organs and glands of the body. She also developed the "Ingham Compression Method of Reflexology." Her two books *Stories the Feet Can Tell* and *Stories the Feet Have Told* are now standard textbooks for reflexology students. She had her own successful practice, and lectured and trained many practitioners in the United States.

Mrs. Doreen E. Bayly, a British nurse, discovered reflexology for herself when she went to visit her sister, a healer in the United States. While there, she met Eunice Ingham and studied with her, returning to Great Britain in the early 1960s. Doreen Bayly managed, despite encountering some opposition at first, to make reflexology known in Great Britain and Europe. She also built up a successful practice, and founded the Bayly School of Reflexology.

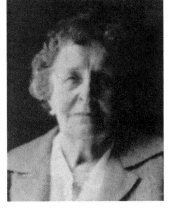

Eunice Ingham is credited as the "mother of reflexology" for mapping out the reflexes on the hands and feet.

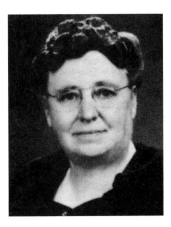

Doreen Bayly, who believed that reflexology worked through electrical impulses in the body.

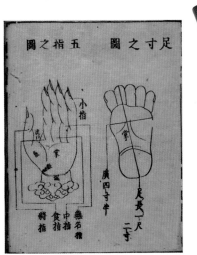

Diagram showing acupuncture points in the hands and feet, from a classic Chinese work in acupuncture literature, the Shisijing Fahui (The enlargement of the fourteen channels), dating back to 1341 by Hua Shou.

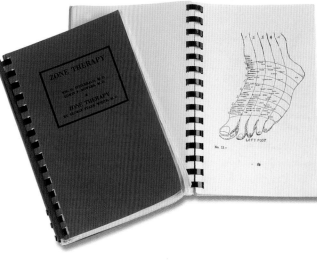

After practicing in hospitals in London and Vienna, Dr. Fitzgerald wrote the highly influential Zone Therapy.

the roots of reflexology

8

Reflexology traces its origins back to traditional Chinese medicine, and it is useful to have an understanding of some of the basic priniciples of this philosophy.

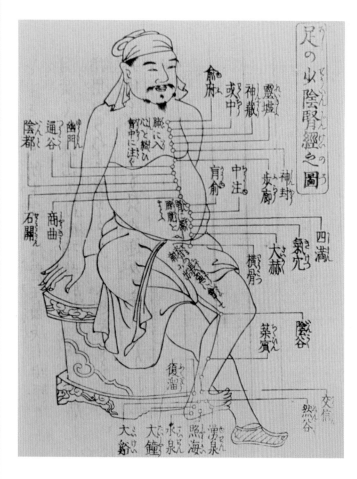

A nineteenth-century Chinese illustration of acupuncture points of the human body.

C hinese philosophy is a vast and complex subject, and it is outside the scope of this book. However, the basis of the philosophy can be roughly broken down into the following:

- Yin and Yang
- Five elements
- The philosophies of the Dao, or Tao, which are often translated as "the path" or "the way of life"
- The Eight Principles. These provide the basic categories for describing the various body disharmonies, such as hot/cold, full/empty, etc.
- Three forms of energy called Qi (pronounced "chee"), Jing, and Shen, which are together called the Three Treasures.

The concept of Yin and Yang is fundamental to understanding Chinese medicine. They are opposites but also complementary. Together they make a whole, but neither is more important than the other. They are two primal forces that can be used to describe anything in the universe, where the ideal balance is depicted in the traditional Yin Yang symbol—the white (Yang) part of the diagram increases as the black (Yin) part decreases. When Yin is at its height, then Yang is at its lowest ebb, and vice versa.

From Yin and Yang, the ancient Chinese developed the theory of the five elements of wood, fire, earth, metal, and water, which they used to describe the cyclic nature of the universe. The laws of the universe cause these elements to interact with each other endlessly: a tree (wood), when burned (fire), produces steam (water) and so on.

Classical Taoism teaches that there is a flow and order in the universe, called Tao, which can be translated simply as the "way of nature." It is never stagnant and it keeps things in the universe balanced and in order. It manifests itself through change of seasons, cycle of life, shifts of power, time, and so forth. Taoism is so called because it shows how to live according to the Tao by going with the flow and not struggling against the tide.

The Eight Principles are one of the basic ways Chinese medicine has to diagnose, using the following eight divisions of symptoms: Yin or Yang, superficial or internal, cold or hot, and deficient or replete.

Traditional Chinese medicine attributes good health to the free flow of Qi energy through the body along energy channels, or meridians, that correspond to organs in the body. When the flow of Qi becomes unbalanced through physical, emotional, or environmental stresses, illness may result. These points can be manipulated through the application of pressure to ensure a well-balanced flow of energy.

Qi is present in every living organism—without it there is no longer life. In Chinese philosophy, as well as many other traditions, everything is related to something else. Nothing truly exists in isolation. Each part of the person is interconnected with the other parts of the body, which is interconnected with the mind, and the external environment. Deforestation, the erosion of soil, the changes in greenhouse gases, the lack of time, and so on, all have an effect on our bodies and minds.

In this system, the removal of, let's say, the spleen, does not mean in Eastern terms that the particular person is cured of his or her ailment, because the disease of the spleen could be caused by many factors. For example, the person could worry a lot, have a sweet tooth, and so on. Those factors would also have to be addressed when treating that person to make him or her whole.

The symbol of the Chinese Yin and Yang philosophy demonstrates the complementary nature of two opposing elements. Yin and Yang are in equal proportion and the curved line represents the constant flow of Yang into Yin and vice versa.

Meridians and acupuncture points on the body, shown by a model and charts. Knowledge of the meridians has been passed down to us through ancient Chinese techniques.

elements

Everything on the earth can be classified into one or more of the five elements. These are wood, fire, earth, metal, and water. In traditional Chinese medicine, these five elements form two cycles—the creative cycle and the destructive cycle.

The creative cycle

Wood will burn to create fire, which when it has finished burning produces ashes (earth). Earth contains metals, which when heated will become molten, like water—which is necessary for the growth of plants and wood.

The destructive cycle

Wood destroys earth—the roots of plants and trees can break up the soil. Earth destroys water—its earthen banks contain a pond. Water destroys fire. Fire destroys metal—a metal object will eventually melt when it is placed in the fire. Metal destroys wood—a metal saw or axe can cut a tree down.

The creative element cycle (right). The ancient Chinese theory of the elements is related to the Taoist philosophical beliefs that dominate traditional Chinese culture.

WOOD
LIVER AND GALLBLADDER

WATER
KIDNEYS AND BLADDER

WATER

WOOD

METAL

METAL
LUNGS AND LARGE INTESTINE

In traditional Chinese medicine, the law of the five elements is as follows:

• Wood is associated with the liver and the gallbladder.

• Fire is associated with the heart, pericardium, triple burner (a concept unique to this system of medicine), and small intestine.

• Earth is associated with the spleen and stomach.

• Metal is associated with the lungs and large intestine.

• Water is associated with the kidneys and bladder.

By using the theory of the five elements, one can understand that, for example, when the liver (wood) is tonified, the heart (fire) will also be tonified, while the stomach and spleen (earth) will be sedated. Looking at another example, if the kidneys (water) are sedated, the liver (wood) will also be sedated, and the heart (fire) will be tonified.

This relationship between the five elements and their associated organs helps the practitioner to understand unexpected results when carrying out a reflexology treatment.

The secret to an active, healthy, and happy life lies in ensuring that all of the bodily systems are working in harmony. The theory of the elements can help us to achieve this.

FIRE
HEART, PERICARDIUM, TRIPLE BURNER, AND SMALL INTESTINE

EARTH
SPLEEN AND STOMACH

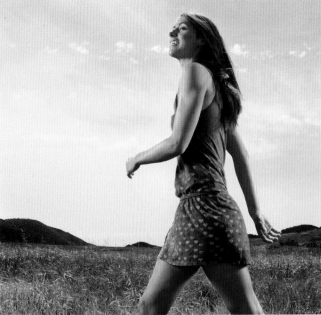

how does reflexology work?

12

The body has five longitudinal zones on each side of the median (or central) line of the body, which run from the tips of the fingers and thumbs, up through the brain, and down to the tips of the toes. These zones can be visualized as longitudinal sections through the body, extending from front to back and containing the internal organs and glands of that section.

T he longitudinal zones or energy channels used in reflexology are considered to be paths along which someone's vital energy, or Qi, flows. Stress, disease, and injury can all lead to congestion along these energy pathways.

Whichever zone or zones an organ occurs in, then the corresponding reflex area will be found within the same zone(s) in the hands or feet. By stimulating the various reflexes on the feet and hands, it is possible to clear away the congestion of toxic deposits that inhibit the flow of the vital force through our bodies, thereby bringing about a state of equilibrium or balance (homeostasis) within the body. This will improve our health and vitality.

*In common with many holistic therapies,
reflexology works on the principle that
energy balance will lead to greater vitality.*

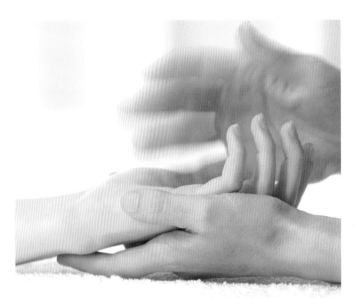

Reflexologists believe that an illness can be a result of an energy blockage in the system; for example, a blockage in the respiratory system could result in the symptoms of the common cold.

Every part of the foot or hand contains reflex areas, which correspond to a part of the body. The feet (soles, tops, and sides) are more commonly used in reflexology than other parts of the body because their reflexes are easier to locate.

Three lateral lines can be used to divide the body at the shoulders, diaphragm, and waist on the soles of the feet and palms of the hand. These act as guidelines, helping to pinpoint more precisely which part of the foot or hand to target with reflexology. Because the hands are much smaller than the feet, the hand guidelines are closer together than the foot guidelines. Similarly, the reflex areas on the hands are concentrated in a smaller area. As a result, they are less detailed (see pages 26–33 for reflex maps of the hands and feet).

Reflexology, being a holistic therapy, uses the principle of the whole being present in each part. No one body part works in isolation; every part works together for the benefit of all. Thus the build-up of toxins in one part of the body eventually leads to different parts having to work harder to compensate for the imbalance in body energies.

Exactly how massaging a reflex can produce a measurable effect on another part of the body is not fully understood. It is, however, accepted that a reflexology treatment has a beneficial effect on the blood circulation and the nervous system.

Acupuncture meridians closely mirror the zones used in reflexology.

Acupuncture meridians and reflexology zones

Similar to the zones in reflexology are the meridians in traditional Chinese medicine. These were discovered as long ago as 2,500 BCE. This system of medicine classifies 1,000 or so acupuncture points into 12 main groups. An imaginary line joins all the acupuncture points belonging to any one of these groups. These lines, known as "meridians," are energy pathways, along which flows the vital life force of Qi or chi.

There are thought to be very close links between the principles of zone therapy (reflexology) and meridian theory (Chinese acupuncture). As with the reflexology zones, the meridians are duplicated on each side of the body, with two central meridians (known as the "governing" and "conception" meridians) running down the front and back of the body along its central or median line.

When there is a build-up of toxins along a certain meridian, this causes a congestion of energy. This congestion will affect the organ associated with that meridian (for example, the lung in the lung meridian), which will suffer a lack of energy. By stimulating one or more acupuncture points on the meridian using reflexology techniques, the congestion is eased, returning the organ to a harmonious state.

The effect of reflexology on the circulatory system

The truth of Eunice Ingham's famous saying, "circulation is life; stagnation is death," can be shown by cutting off the blood supply to even the smallest part of the body. Soon a variety of aches and pains occur, and the color starts changing. If the blockage continues, the affected part will eventually die.

We all know that our hands and feet will respond to cold conditions by starting to ache; this is because cold has the effect of reducing the blood supply. Organs and glands that do not receive a sufficiently rich supply of blood malfunction and lose their balancing qualities. The body then slowly stops being a harmonious unit.

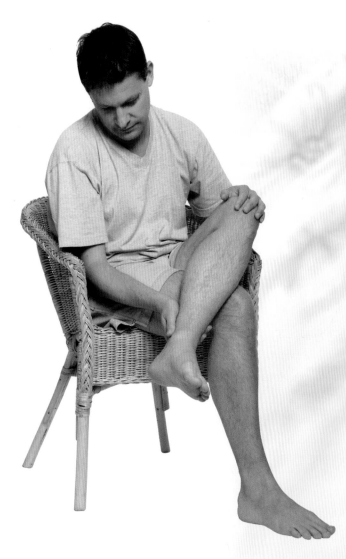

Exposed and hardworking, the feet themselves are particularly vulnerable to circulatory disorders.

Tension has the effect of restricting blood flow, causing high or low blood pressure. High blood pressure can cause thickening of the blood vessel walls. Materials build up, coating the inside of the arteries, and this is called hardening of the arteries, or arteriosclerosis. When the blood flow is reduced because of the build-up in the artery, the kidney releases the hormone renin, which further increases blood pressure.

Reflexology causes the body to become more relaxed. This facilitates a sufficiently rich supply of blood to the organs and glands, enabling them to start functioning in a more harmonious state.

14

The effect of reflexology on the nervous system

The nerves, which are cord-like structures, convey impulses from the central nervous system to other parts of the body. By this type of communication, they are able to coordinate the function of the organs and the various body parts to enable them to work in equilibrium with one another.

Tension can put pressure on various nerves, causing messages to the organs to be impaired. This often means that the organ will not function as it should. Most of us have had some personal experience of this—tension headaches, for example, are familiar to many.

Reflexology stimulates thousands of nerve endings, and thereby encourages the opening and clearing of neural pathways. Reflexology also reduces tension, and so aids the nervous system.

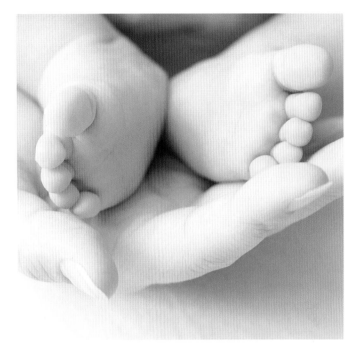

Reflexology can be used to treat specific disorders and anyone, from infants to older people, can benefit from its relaxing effects.

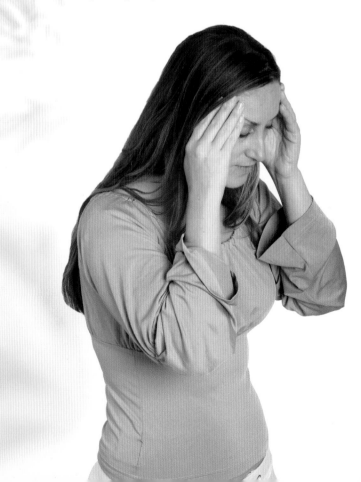

Tension headache is a common condition that causes misery for many people; the answer could lie in a rebalancing of bodily energies.

Benefits and caution

A large proportion, approximately 75 percent, of disorders and diseases are brought about by external influences, such as stress and lifestyle factors. People react to these stresses and tensions in various ways. One person may experience backaches, another cardiovascular problems, another may become more nervous.

However, anyone who is willing to accept responsibility for their own well-being can benefit from a reflexology treatment. Reflexology does not discriminate—anyone, from babies right up to the elderly—can gain relief from it.

By stimulating the elimination of waste materials from the body, or improving the circulation, it is possible to speed up the healing process, thereby normalizing bodily functions.

Most disorders will benefit from a reflexology treatment; however, it is unsuitable for some (see page 65 for details).

body systems

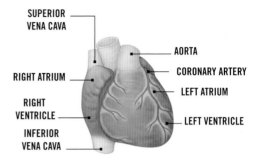

The circulatory system of an adult contains 12½ pints (6 liters) of blood, and the heart is powerful enough to pump it all around the body.

Reflexology is a holistic therapy; among other things, this means that all of the following systems need to be taken into account, and they must work harmoniously together to produce a physically and mentally healthy person.

Muscular system

Muscles are composed of tissue that can be contracted so that movement can occur. They convert energy from food and respiration into physical movement, usually in response to signals from the brain and the nervous system. There are three main types of muscle tissue:

Skeletal: This type of muscle is under the mind's conscious control, and it will respond to nervous signals by controlling the movement of the relevant skeletal bone (for example, the biceps pulls on the humerus to elevate the upper arm).

Smooth: This is found in the intestines and the lining of organs and is not under conscious control.

Cardiac: This is a special type of involuntary muscle and is found only in the heart.

Circulatory system

The heart, an organ about the size of a clenched fist, is situated in the thorax. The right ventricle pumps deoxygenated blood to the lungs, where carbon dioxide and oxygen are exchanged. Oxygenated blood returns to the left atrium. This is known as the pulmonary circulation. The left ventricle pumps the oxygenated blood and nutrition to all the other parts of the body, returning via the vena cava with the waste products that have to be filtered and excreted. Carbon dioxide is also returned to the heart by the systemic circulatory system, where, after being pumped through the heart chambers, it enters the pulmonary circulatory system and the process starts again.

Nervous system

The nervous system is made up of two parts:

The central nervous system: This consists of the brain and the spinal cord.

The peripheral nervous system: This carries information from various parts of the body, through the relevant sensory nerves to the central nervous system. It carries out instructions through the efferent motor nerves (nerve cells that carry impulses away from the central nervous system to related parts of the body). The nerves are made up of thousands of long, thin nerve fibers.

Respiratory system

The human respiratory system is made up of the nose and mouth, the pharynx and larynx in the throat, and the windpipe, or trachea. The trachea then divides into two bronchi, which enter the lungs. The bronchi subdivide into smaller bronchioles, at the end of which are the alveolar sacs, containing the individual alveoli. This is where gaseous exchange occurs.

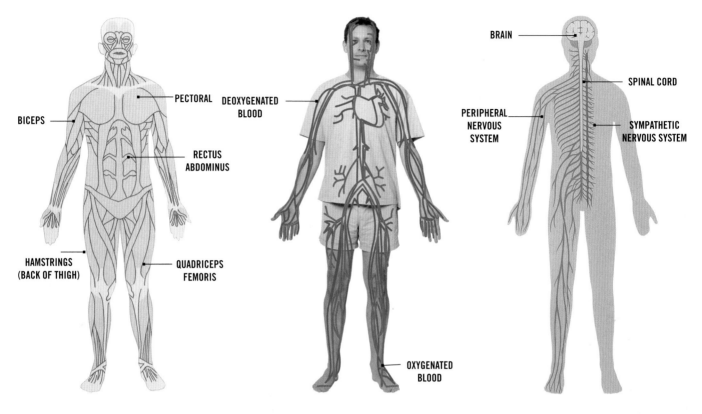

BICEPS

PECTORAL

DEOXYGENATED BLOOD

RECTUS ABDOMINUS

HAMSTRINGS (BACK OF THIGH)

QUADRICEPS FEMORIS

OXYGENATED BLOOD

BRAIN

SPINAL CORD

PERIPHERAL NERVOUS SYSTEM

SYMPATHETIC NERVOUS SYSTEM

Consciously controlled skeletal muscles are responsible for the large movements the body makes.

The circulatory system contains the heart itself as well as the blood circulation network.

The central nervous system, together with the peripheral system, controls movement in the body.

Endocrine system

The endocrine system consists of ductless glands, which produce and secrete hormones directly into the bloodstream. These hormones are carried in the blood until they affect those organs that are sensitive to them. The endocrine glands include the pituitary gland, which is found in the brain. It controls the function of the thyroid, adrenals, and the reproductive glands (the ovaries and testes). The activity of the pituitary is regulated by the hypothalamus, which is found just above the pituitary.

Urinary system

The urinary system consists of the kidneys, situated on either side of the spine. They filter the blood as well as regulate the composition and volume of the body fluids by eliminating what cannot be reused—for example, salts, waste products, and excess water. The kidneys are connected to the bladder by the ureter tubes. Urine continuously drains out of the kidneys into the ureters and into the bladder. The bladder wall contains sensory nerve endings that send messages to the brain, alerting the person when the bladder needs to be emptied.

Reproductive system

Most of the male reproductive anatomy is external. The two testes hang in scrotal sacs. Two long convoluted tubes called the epididymis, one on each side, are attached to the testes. These allow the sperm, which have been produced in the testes, to ripen. The epididymis then opens into the vas deferens, another long tube on each side of the body, which is joined to the seminal vesicles. The seminal vesicles act as a storage place for mature sperm before they are released into the urethra. The female reproductive organs consist of the ovaries, Fallopian tubes, the uterus, and the vagina.

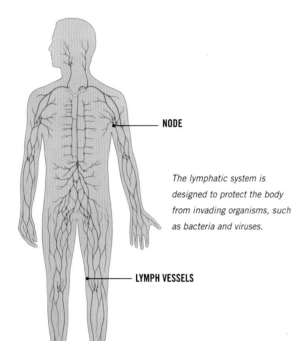

NODE

The lymphatic system is designed to protect the body from invading organisms, such as bacteria and viruses.

LYMPH VESSELS

Lymphatic system

This is our defense system for protecting the body from bacteria and other organisms. Lymph is transported by the lymphatic system, along which lymph nodes are situated at intervals. The lymph nodes contain a system of narrow channels along which the lymph drains. Along the walls of these channels, large phagocytes (cells that engulf particles) surround bacteria, other harmful substances, and dead cells from the lymph. Large lymph nodes are found in the neck, under the arms, in the breast, and in the groin. The spleen plays an important part in the lymphatic system, producing lymphocytes (white blood cells), and helping to break down and recycle hemoglobin from old blood cells.

Digestive system

Digestion starts in the mouth. Food is chewed and mixed with saliva, which contains enzymes that make a start on the process of breaking larger molecules down into smaller, more easily absorbed, molecules. The saliva also lubricates the food, making it softer and easier to swallow. The ingested food then enters the esophagus and travels to the stomach. Here, it is churned and mixed with the stomach acids that change the food substances into a state that is more easily absorbed. The mixture then enters the small intestine and the large intestine, where further breakdown and absorption take place. The liver, gallbladder and pancreas are also important in the digestion process.

Skeletal system

The bones give the body support and protect the internal glands and organs. They also give the body its shape, and they regulate minerals, particularly calcium, phosphorous, copper, and cobalt. Healthy bone marrow is vital, because it manufactures red and white blood cells as well as platelets.

Sensory system

The sense organs allow the body to be aware of its environment. When a sensory cell is stimulated, electrical impulses are sent along nerve pathways to the brain. Once the

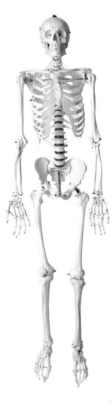

As well as providing the structure for our bodies, the bones of our skeletal system contain marrow, which plays a vital role in the production of white blood cells to fight infection, red blood cells to carry oxygen, and platelets, which help the clotting process.

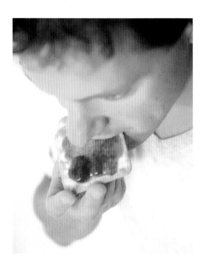

The human sense of smell, while not as acute as that possessed by some other mammals, has many uses. It seems to have a profound effect on the emotions, as well as our sense of taste.

signals arrive at the appropriate part of the brain, they are interpreted as sight, sound, pain, and so on. The following organs are part of the sensory system:

The skin: This is a waterproof protective layer around the body that protects us from shock and infection. It regulates our body temperature and is sensitive to touch, temperature, pressure, and pain. The skin also has an important excretory function.

The eyes: These complex organs allow us to see by the use of the cornea (which aids focusing), a lens, an adjustable iris with the pupil at its center, and the retina, which contains millions of light-sensitive cells. The visual information is then carried to the brain by nerves.

The ears: The ear is made up of three parts. The outer ear picks up sound and sends it to the middle ear, which contains the eardrum and three small bones. These magnify the sound before sending it to the inner ear, which has the cochlea, a snail shell-like structure containing microscopic nerve cells, each one of which is sensitive to a certain vibration. The vibrations produce an electric current, which is carried by the auditory nerve to the brain, where it is decoded into what we describe as "sound" or "noise."

The inner ear is also responsible for balance. The three semicircular canals are filled with a fluid that sends messages to the brain by means of tiny hairs and nerves in the ear, allowing the person to maintain their equilibrium.

The nose: The nose has numerous functions. Its primary use is in breathing, during which process it filters out particles from the air through the nasal hairs and mucous before the air enters the lungs. The olfactory organs, which are sensitive to smell, are found in the upper regions of the nasal cavity. When chemical molecules stimulate these organs, nerve endings will send the messages to the olfactory part of the brain, where they are decoded. The senses of smell and taste are closely linked.

The tongue: The tongue contains various muscles going in different directions, which allows it to be a highly mobile organ. This is important in the chewing process, as well as in swallowing and speech. The tongue is also highly sensitive to temperature, touch, and, of course, taste. Taste buds are located on the surface of the tongue among 9,000 or so tiny projections, which are called papillae.

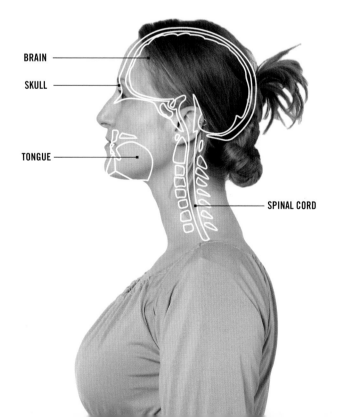

BRAIN

SKULL

TONGUE

SPINAL CORD

reflexology and everyone

Everyone can enjoy, and benefit from, a reflexology treatment. Whether you are young or old, male or female, the treatment will have some effect.

R eflexology is suitable and safe for all ages and may bring relief for a wide range of acute and chronic conditions. Reflexology treats the whole person by looking at the balance between the body, emotions, and environment. A reflexology treatment can therefore combat a number of disorders, or disease, by bringing the mind, body, and spirit back to a more harmonious state. You do not have to be ill or physically uncomfortable to experience the benefits it can offer. Reflexology has the ability to make people feel better by simply removing stress from the whole body and generating a sense of deep relaxation. Because people frequently struggle to find the time to relax properly, almost everyone can benefit from treatment.

Babies
Babies appear to respond particularly well to a gentle reflexology session. It can relax a baby after birth as well as strengthen the special bond between parents and babies. It has been shown to be effective in helping babies sleep, aiding colic, and helping crying babies and their mothers unwind.

Children
Reflexology is a great way for parents or carers to connect with children, especially when they are ill and less able to

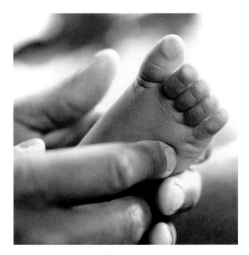

Reflexology provides a wonderful way to connect with babies and a little goes a long way. When applied very gently, it can produce many benefits, including the relief of common ailments, such as diarrhea and colic.

communicate. Children can also learn self-help techniques, which is invaluable in teaching them about the links between their mind and body and self-reliance. Children are often more receptive to new experiences, and, therefore, natural remedies, than adults. Older children may benefit when hormonal changes take place around puberty, and reflexology can be used to destress before an important exam, aiding relaxation.

Women
Many of the disharmonies and disorders that may occur during a woman's fertile life respond well to reflexology therapy. Reflexology may help maintain regular cycles, reduce painful periods or heavy periods, relieve PMS, and support women through the menopause.

Reflexology is especially beneficial for pregnant women after their first trimester. It can help with all pregnancy-related problems, and it has been claimed that it can shorten labor times and increase the strength and efficacy of contractions. It also gives mothers and babies the relaxation they need.

Adults

Reflexology has helped couples conceive, where there are no physical problems. Some HIV and drug rehabilitation centers now offer reflexology to their clients as well, and the stress-relieving benefits of the procedure have been shown to be effective in helping people with mental health problems. Reflexology is now used in many hospices to relieve physical symptoms, such as pain, and also to provide the opportunity for loved ones to maintain a therapeutic emotional connection.

Older people

Reflexology benefits the elderly by improving circulation and may help to increase mobility. It also offers the potential to counter pain and ease the physical effects of aging, such as aching joints and incontinence. The lack of physical contact and loneliness that can be associated with old age can be ameliorated by reflexology, helping people simply to feel better in themselves. Hand massage has been shown to help calm down elderly people with dementia.

Reflexology and medicine

Increasingly, reflexology is being offered as a mainstream treatment. However, it should be stressed that reflexologists—unless they are licensed physicians—do not practice medicine. They should never try to diagnose a disease, or to prescribe or adjust a client's medication, and should advise a client to see their medical practitioner when necessary. Responsible reflexologists do not treat specific diseases, although by returning the body to a more harmonious state, a treatment can benefit a number of disorders.

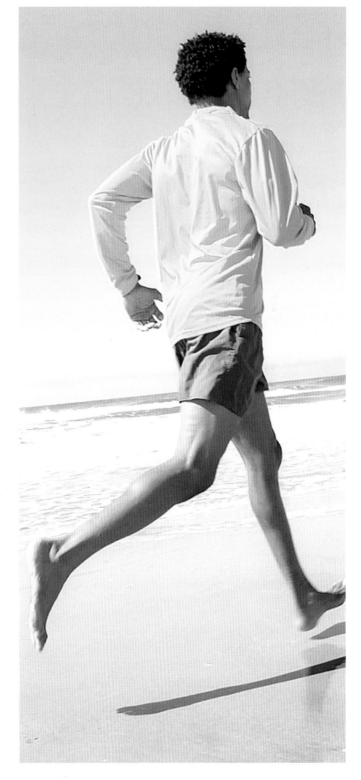

Reflexology can benefit everyone by reducing stress and increasing a sense of well-being and harmony.

introduction to reflex maps

One of the most important parts of reflexology is a thorough understanding of how the feet and hands can be seen as a map of the whole body. The right foot represents the right side of the body, the inside of the foot representing the right half of the spine. The left foot represents the left side of the body, with the inside representing the left half of the spine.

It is said that all the organs of the body are represented on the hands and the feet. This is also thought to be true of the iris of the eye (iridology), the ear (ear acupuncture and ear reflexology), and the head.

The hands and feet are, therefore, like small maps of the whole body. All the organs, glands, and various body parts are imaged on the feet and hands in almost the same arrangement as in the body. Reflex areas are found on the soles, sides, and tops of the feet. The hands also contain reflex areas on their palms, sides, and tops.

The reflexes in the hands are in a similar position to those of the feet, although many of the areas are more condensed than in the feet, with the exception of the fingers. The fingers, however, still contain the same reflexes as the toes and they are in similar positions.

The reason that the reflex maps of the feet and hands are so similar is due to our evolutionary ancestors, who in the past walked on all fours. Although we evolved into bipeds and our legs got stronger and longer and our arms weaker and perhaps shorter, the relative positions of the reflexes stayed roughly the same. This idea can be taken further than just feet and hands. For example, if you wanted to work on somebody's knee, but were unable to do so for some reason, then the elbow could be used. Likewise the shoulder could be used for working the hip, the wrist used for the ankle, and vice versa.

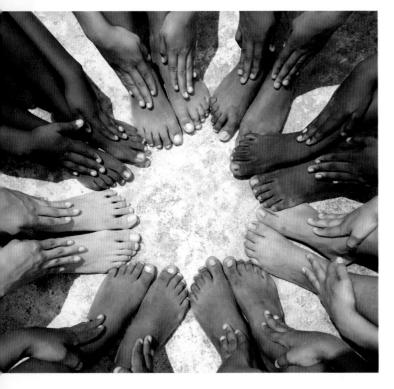

There are so many nerve endings, bones, and muscles in the foot that massage can have a very positive effect on our feelings of well-being.

FOOT AND HAND ZONES

Although reflexology is an ancient art, Dr. William H. Fitzgerald was the first person to describe how the longitudinal zones of the body correspond to the zones of the feet and the hands.

Each finger and each toe falls into one of the five zones to be found on that side of the body, and points in that zone can be used to treat the related areas.

LONGITUDINAL ZONES

The body is divided in two lengthwise by the median line; there are five longitudinal zones on each half of the body.

23

The zones

The hand and the foot are divided into five longitudinal zones. The left hand represents the left-hand side of the body and the right hand represents the right-hand side of the body. Each reflexology zone contains one finger and one toe. Zone 1 contains the thumb and big toe, and all the organs and tissues in that longitudinal zone, zone 2 contains the second finger and toe, and so on until we get to the little toe and finger in zone 5.

When trying to work out and remember the various reflexes, you need to think about the various organs and where they are in the body. Those found in the center of the body, such as the brain, neck, heart, and spine, are all found in zone 1. There are, however, a few exceptions. The bladder, for example, is found in zone 1 for the feet and in zone 3 in the hands. Zone 5 contains the limbs and other organs situated on the sides of the body. The eyes are found in zones 2 and 3 in both the feet and hands and the ears in zones 3 and 4.

It is worth noting that the right side of the brain is located in the right foot and hand, and the left side in the left foot and hand. The zones do not cross in the brain, as the nervous system does. Reflexologists believe that any condition that obstructs the energy flow through a given zone will impede the healthy functioning of the body parts along it. By working any point of the zones, the hands and feet can release tension and restore equilibrium to the entire zone and so to the body.

reflex maps and anatomy

The foot and hand have similar basic structures. The feet bear the whole of the body weight. The heel, the base of the big toe, and the base of the little toe form a kind of three-dimensional arch that supports the body. The hand, which does not have to bear any body weight, is more delicate, with long, easily mobile fingers. Understanding these structures can help you to locate the reflex areas more accurately.

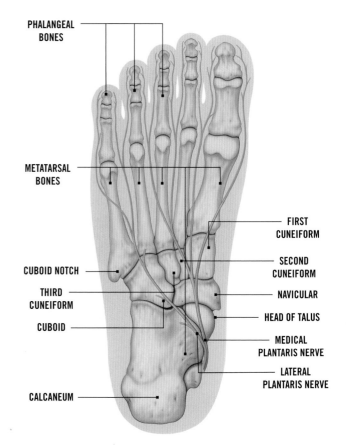

PHALANGEAL BONES

METATARSAL BONES

FIRST CUNEIFORM

SECOND CUNEIFORM

CUBOID NOTCH

THIRD CUNEIFORM

NAVICULAR

CUBOID

HEAD OF TALUS

MEDICAL PLANTARIS NERVE

LATERAL PLANTARIS NERVE

CALCANEUM

Anatomy of the foot

The many muscles, the numerous ligaments, and the bones that make up the foot create systems of fulcrums and levers, which make the feet strong and flexible.

- Each foot is made up of 26 bones.
- Each toe is made up of three bones (except the big toe, which has only two). These bones are called the phalanges.
- Below the phalanges are the five metatarsals. These link each toe to the other bones of the foot.
- The cuboid bone is found under the little and fourth toe metatarsals.
- The side protrusion on the cuboid bone is called the cuboid notch. The three smaller cuneiforms are found under the big toe and the second and third toes. The navicular is positioned below the cuneiforms.

- The calcaneum (heel bone) and the talus are found in the heel region of the foot.
- The cuboid, cuneiforms, navicular, calcaneum, and talus, grouped together, are known as the tarsal bones.

Anatomy of the hand

- Each hand is made up of 27 bones.
- The thumb is made up of two phalanges and the four fingers each have three phalanges.
- At the base of each of the phalanges is a metacarpal bone. The five metacarpal bones form the palm of the hand. The eight carpal bones are made up of the trapezium, which is

under the thumb metacarpal; the trapezoid, under the index finger metacarpal; the capitate, under the middle finger metacarpal; and the hamate, under the fourth and fifth metacarpals. The scaphoid, lunate, triquetral, and pisiform are found in the wrist.

• The mobility of the carpal bones, along with the associated muscles, tendons, and ligaments, which also keep the bones in place, make the hand a very flexible and precise tool.

Reflexology areas and anatomy

As explained on pages 23–24, the foot and hand can be divided into areas that mirror the body.

• The head and neck are represented by the toes and fingers. The right foot or hand represents the right side of the head with its associated organs, and the left foot or hand the left side of the head with its various organs.

• The thoracic and upper abdominal area (from the shoulders to the diaphragm, most of the stomach, and part of the kidneys) is represented by the ball of the foot, or more precisely the area between the bottom of the phalanges to the bottom of the metatarsal bones. This area is between the bottom of the phalanges and the bottom of the metacarpal bones on the hand. The line at the bottom of the metatarsal bones is often referred to as the waistline, and can be more easily located by running a horizontal line across the foot from the cuboid notch. On the hand, this line is found at the bottom of the metacarpal bones.

• The lower abdominal area (from the lower part of the stomach and kidneys to the pelvis) is represented on the foot by the area between the waistline and the pelvic line. This is located by connecting the inner and outer anklebone protrusions (malleoli), which run under the foot. Thus, the reflexes of the abdomen and pelvis are found over the tarsal bones and around the anklebones. On the hand, this area is found over the carpal bones.

• The pelvic area (the knee, leg, hip, and lower back reflexes)

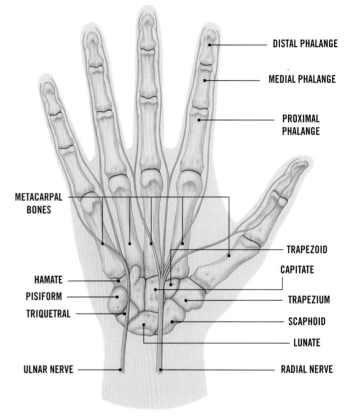

DISTAL PHALANGE

MEDIAL PHALANGE

PROXIMAL PHALANGE

METACARPAL BONES

HAMATE

PISIFORM

TRIQUETRAL

ULNAR NERVE

TRAPEZOID

CAPITATE

TRAPEZIUM

SCAPHOID

LUNATE

RADIAL NERVE

is represented by the heel, running from the pelvic line to the rear of the heel, and on the top of both hands on the outer side of zone 5 (the area below the little finger).

• The reproductive area is represented by different parts of the ankle or wrist.

• The spine is represented by the instep and the outside edge of the thumb. The curve of a person's spine will closely resemble the natural sweep of the instep.

• The arms and legs are represented by the outer edges of the foot and on the little finger side of the hand.

• The reflexes for the breast and lymphatic system are on the top of the foot and the top of the hand.

foot maps: the soles

26

The soles of the feet contain many thousands of reflexes, which can be grouped together according to which body part they affect.

E ach area contains many reflex points in a similar way to pins in a pincushion. You can see from these diagrams that the areas closely relate to the position of the organs. The body itself can be divided into four clearly delineated horizontal zones on the soles of the feet: the head and neck areas are found on the toes; the thoracic area (from the shoulders down to the diaphragm) is found on the ball of the foot; the abdominal area (from the diaphragm down to the pelvic area) is on the arch; and the pelvic area is on the heel.

The right sole

The right sole has reflex areas that correspond to the body's right-hand side. For example, the liver reflex site is much larger on this sole because the liver sits on the right side of the body.

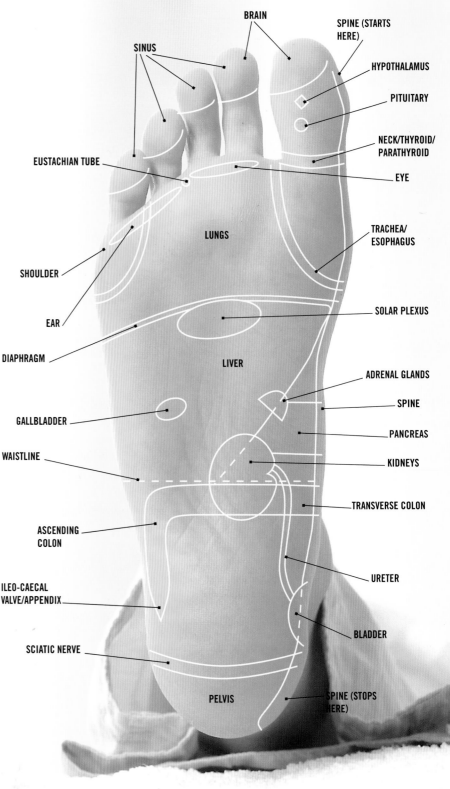

BRAIN

SPINE (STARTS HERE)

SINUS

HYPOTHALAMUS

PITUITARY

NECK/THYROID/ PARATHYROID

EYE

EUSTACHIAN TUBE

TRACHEA/ ESOPHAGUS

LUNGS

SHOULDER

SOLAR PLEXUS

EAR

DIAPHRAGM

LIVER

ADRENAL GLANDS

SPINE

GALLBLADDER

PANCREAS

WAISTLINE

KIDNEYS

TRANSVERSE COLON

ASCENDING COLON

URETER

ILEO-CAECAL VALVE/APPENDIX

BLADDER

SCIATIC NERVE

PELVIS

SPINE (STOPS HERE)

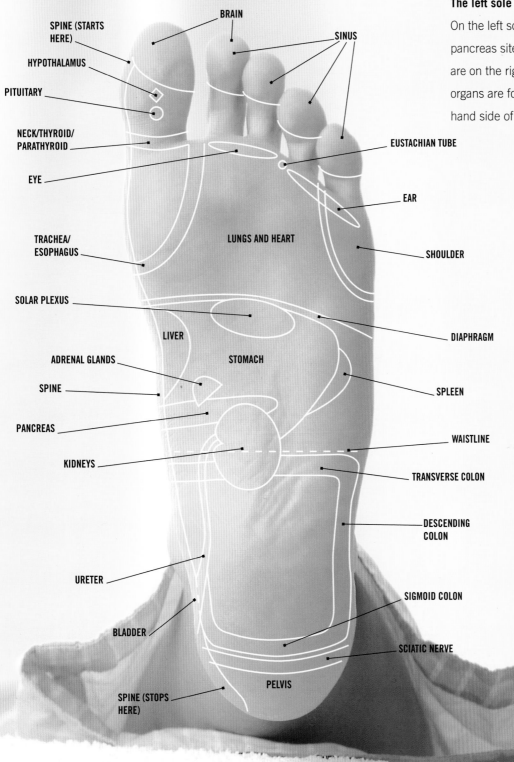

SPINE (STARTS HERE)

BRAIN

SINUS

HYPOTHALAMUS

PITUITARY

NECK/THYROID/ PARATHYROID

EUSTACHIAN TUBE

EYE

EAR

TRACHEA/ ESOPHAGUS

LUNGS AND HEART

SHOULDER

SOLAR PLEXUS

DIAPHRAGM

LIVER

ADRENAL GLANDS

STOMACH

SPINE

SPLEEN

PANCREAS

WAISTLINE

KIDNEYS

TRANSVERSE COLON

DESCENDING COLON

URETER

SIGMOID COLON

BLADDER

SCIATIC NERVE

DESCENDING COLON

PELVIS

SPINE (STOPS HERE)

The left sole

On the left sole, the stomach and pancreas sites are larger than they are on the right sole because these organs are found more on the left-hand side of the body.

foot maps: the tops and sides

There are fewer reflexes on the tops and sides of the feet because the tops are more bony than the soles, making it harder to connect to the reflexes.

Inside

The natural curve of the inside of each foot represents the spine. The big toe area corresponds to the neck, the area from the shoulders to waistline lies on the ball of the foot, the area between the waist and the pelvis is found in the foot's arch, while the base of the heel corresponds to the tailbone.

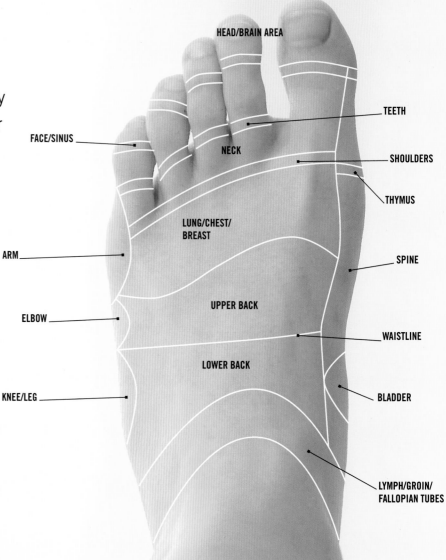

HEAD/BRAIN AREA

TEETH

FACE/SINUS

NECK

SHOULDERS

THYMUS

LUNG/CHEST/
BREAST

ARM

SPINE

UPPER BACK

ELBOW

WAISTLINE

LOWER BACK

KNEE/LEG

BLADDER

LYMPH/GROIN/
FALLOPIAN TUBES

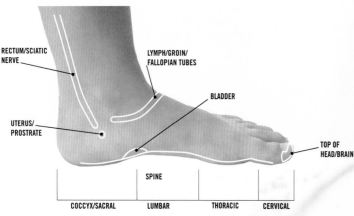

RECTUM/SCIATIC
NERVE

LYMPH/GROIN/
FALLOPIAN TUBES

BLADDER

UTERUS/
PROSTRATE

TOP OF
HEAD/BRAIN

SPINE

COCCYX/SACRAL   LUMBAR   THORACIC   CERVICAL

Tops of the feet

The top of the right foot corresponds to the right side of the body and the top of the left foot the left side. Most of the reflexes found on the soles are also found on the top of the feet with the exception of the circulatory system and the breasts. The upper back and its organs are found above the waistline on both feet. The face/sinus area is a ring found on each toe but the neck area ring only occurs on the four smaller toes.

Outside

The outer edge of the foot corresponds to the outer parts of the body—limbs, joints, and ligaments. The area around the ankle corresponds to the pelvic area and reproductive organs. The outer ankle contains the ovary/testicle reflex points.

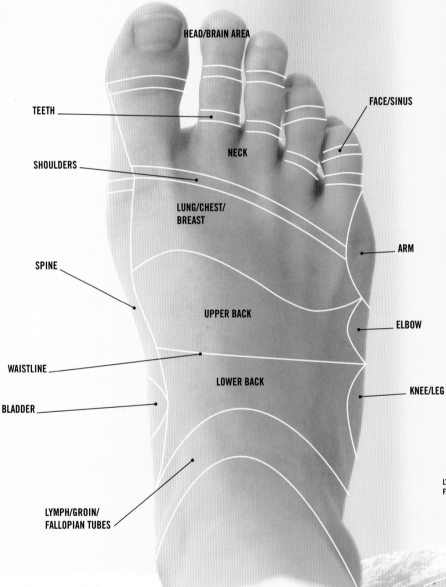

HEAD/BRAIN AREA

FACE/SINUS

TEETH

NECK

SHOULDERS

LUNG/CHEST/BREAST

ARM

SPINE

UPPER BACK

ELBOW

WAISTLINE

LOWER BACK

KNEE/LEG

BLADDER

LYMPH/GROIN/FALLOPIAN TUBES

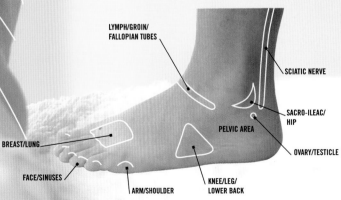

LYMPH/GROIN/FALLOPIAN TUBES

SCIATIC NERVE

SACRO-ILEAC/HIP

PELVIC AREA

BREAST/LUNG

OVARY/TESTICLE

FACE/SINUSES

ARM/SHOULDER

KNEE/LEG/LOWER BACK

hand maps: the palms

30

Hand maps work in exactly the same way as the foot maps, except that the reflexes are more condensed and are consequently less obvious to find.

O n the whole, the reflexes in the hand occupy similar positions to those on the foot. The spine reflex area runs from the outside edge of the thumb, down the palm until it meets the wrist. The tops of the fingers represent the head and the area closest to the wrist represents the tailbone.

The left palm

The reflex areas on the left palm relate to the left side of the body. The spleen reflex is only found on the left palm. The reflexes for the digestive and genitourinary systems of the body are located in the lower part of the hand underneath the diaphragm line.

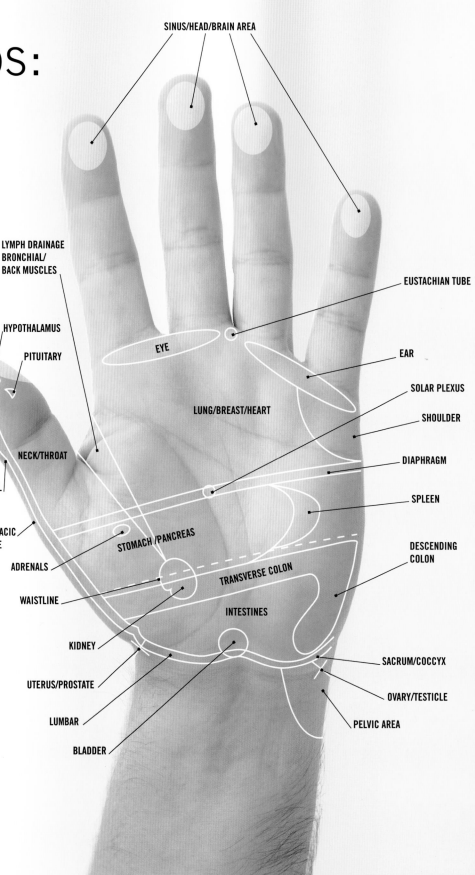

SINUS/HEAD/BRAIN AREA

LYMPH DRAINAGE BRONCHIAL/ BACK MUSCLES

HYPOTHALAMUS

PITUITARY

BRAIN/ HEAD

NECK/THROAT

CERVICAL SPINE

THORACIC SPINE

ADRENALS

WAISTLINE

KIDNEY

UTERUS/PROSTATE

LUMBAR

BLADDER

EYE

LUNG/BREAST/HEART

STOMACH /PANCREAS

TRANSVERSE COLON

INTESTINES

EUSTACHIAN TUBE

EAR

SOLAR PLEXUS

SHOULDER

DIAPHRAGM

SPLEEN

DESCENDING COLON

SACRUM/COCCYX

OVARY/TESTICLE

PELVIC AREA

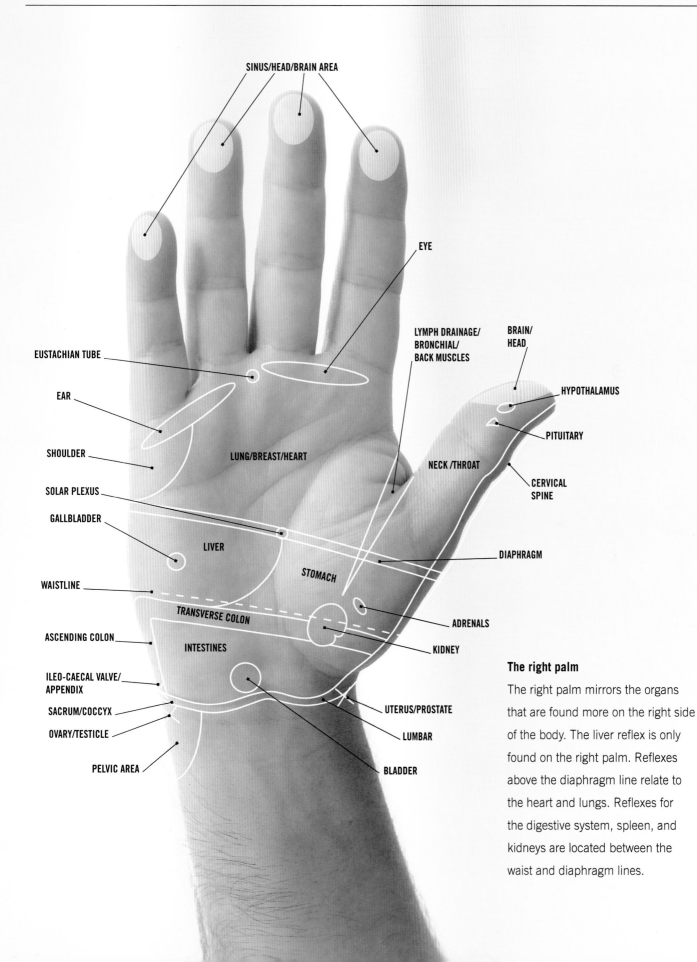

SINUS/HEAD/BRAIN AREA

EYE

LYMPH DRAINAGE/
BRONCHIAL/
BACK MUSCLES

BRAIN/
HEAD

EUSTACHIAN TUBE

HYPOTHALAMUS

EAR

PITUITARY

NECK /THROAT

SHOULDER

CERVICAL
SPINE

LUNG/BREAST/HEART

SOLAR PLEXUS

GALLBLADDER

DIAPHRAGM

LIVER

WAISTLINE

STOMACH

TRANSVERSE COLON

ADRENALS

ASCENDING COLON

INTESTINES

KIDNEY

ILEO-CAECAL VALVE/
APPENDIX

SACRUM/COCCYX

UTERUS/PROSTATE

OVARY/TESTICLE

LUMBAR

PELVIC AREA

BLADDER

The right palm

The right palm mirrors the organs
that are found more on the right side
of the body. The liver reflex is only
found on the right palm. Reflexes
above the diaphragm line relate to
the heart and lungs. Reflexes for
the digestive system, spleen, and
kidneys are located between the
waist and diaphragm lines.

hand maps: the tops

As with the tops of the feet, the tops of the hand are bony, which makes it harder to connect to the reflexes, and the reflex areas tend to be less defined.

T he head is again represented by the tips of the fingers but the area by the wrist contains the reflexes for the lymph glands, groin, and Fallopian tubes. This area wraps around the wrist to form a bracelet.

Top of the left hand

Like the palm, the reflexes on the top of the left hand relate to the left side of the body. The outer edge of the hand corresponds to the outer part of the body from the shoulder and arm all the way down to the knee, leg, and hip regions.

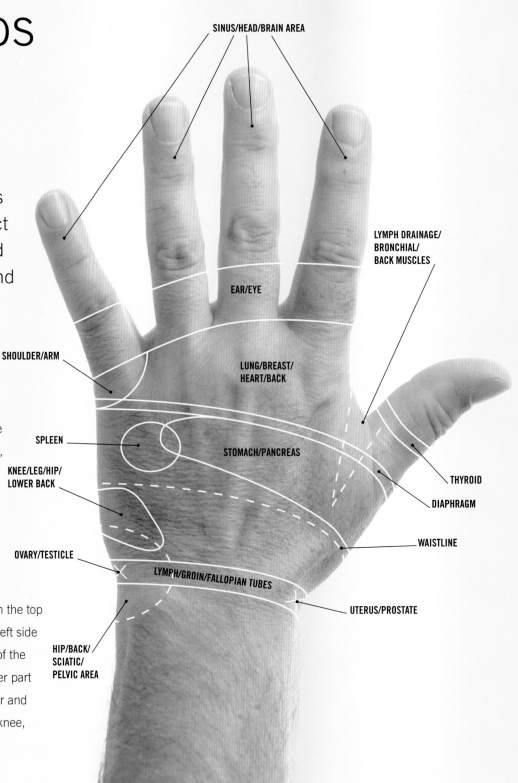

SINUS/HEAD/BRAIN AREA

LYMPH DRAINAGE/
BRONCHIAL/
BACK MUSCLES

EAR/EYE

SHOULDER/ARM

LUNG/BREAST/
HEART/BACK

SPLEEN

STOMACH/PANCREAS

THYROID

KNEE/LEG/HIP/
LOWER BACK

DIAPHRAGM

WAISTLINE

OVARY/TESTICLE

LYMPH/GROIN/FALLOPIAN TUBES

UTERUS/PROSTATE

HIP/BACK/
SCIATIC/
PELVIC AREA

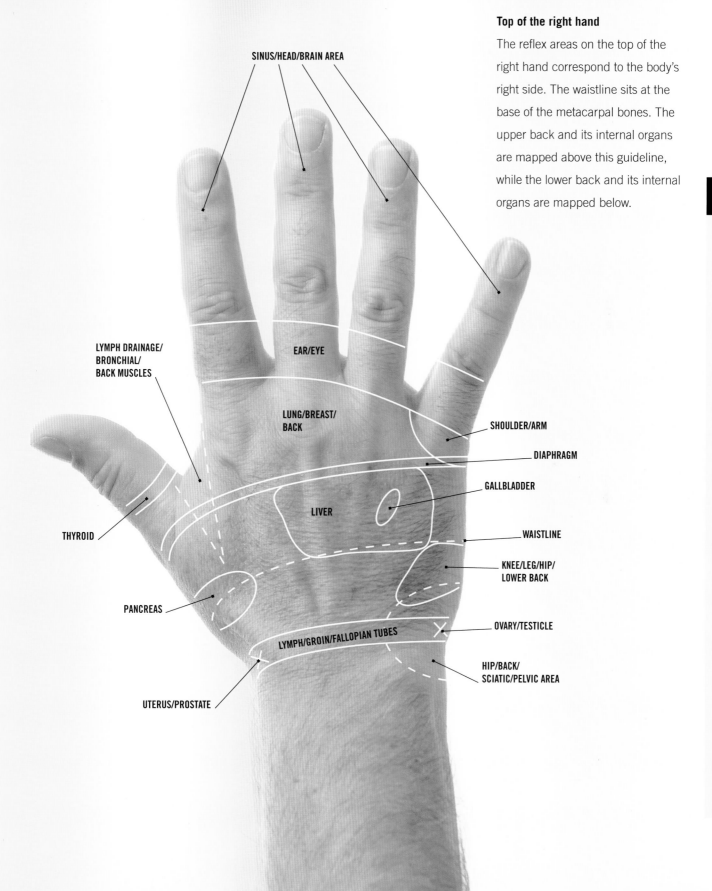

SINUS/HEAD/BRAIN AREA

Top of the right hand

The reflex areas on the top of the right hand correspond to the body's right side. The waistline sits at the base of the metacarpal bones. The upper back and its internal organs are mapped above this guideline, while the lower back and its internal organs are mapped below.

33

LYMPH DRAINAGE/
BRONCHIAL/
BACK MUSCLES

EAR/EYE

LUNG/BREAST/
BACK

SHOULDER/ARM

DIAPHRAGM

GALLBLADDER

LIVER

THYROID

WAISTLINE

KNEE/LEG/HIP/
LOWER BACK

PANCREAS

OVARY/TESTICLE

LYMPH/GROIN/FALLOPIAN TUBES

HIP/BACK/
SCIATIC/PELVIC AREA

UTERUS/PROSTATE

taking care of your hands and feet

Now that we know the whole body is mapped on the feet and hands, and that the body parts are all interrelated, it is easy to see why caring for your hands and feet will affect your whole being.

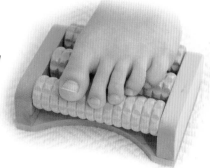

Foot rollers are designed to revive tired feet and improve circulation around the arch and ball of the foot. They are great for massaging, improving circulation, and stimulating the reflexology points.

Feet

Your feet take a great deal of strain. By the time you reach your 50th birthday, it is estimated that they will have carried you around the circumference of the world more than three times. Their functioning is so carefully balanced that just losing a big toe would require time to learn to walk again, because the big toe is fundamental for balance and propelling us forward.

This is why what you wear on your feet is really important. If you continue to wear shoes that fit poorly and do not allow the toes to lie flat, then eventually the toes, which contain some of the smallest bones in the body, will be damaged. The energy along the toes will become compromised and

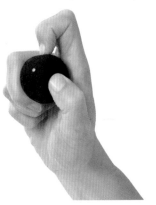

An effective way to develop hand strength is by squeezing a squash ball. Do as many repetitions as possible, building the number up over time.

you may start having headaches, sinus problems, and reproductive difficulties, to name but a few.

Shoes with heels, especially if they are over 2 inches (5 cm high), will affect the feet and posture. They do not allow the toes to lie flat and straight, resulting in metatarsal damage. High-heeled shoes can also shorten calf muscles, and they can cause compression in the lower back, thus causing neck and back pain. Likewise, while less restrictive, not all sandals have the support needed for walking on hard surfaces or for long distances.

Keeping your shoes on for a few hours can create a perfect environment for bacterial and fungal infections. Feet produce warmth and moisture through sweat, and this can lead to infections, such as athlete's foot, as well as bad odor, fissures, cracked skin, and itching. If you are susceptible to fungal infections or have odorous feet, it is worth using a foot powder to absorb the sweat and wearing socks made of natural fibers, because these are better at absorbing the moisture.

People often forget that feet continue to change size and shape throughout the course of their lives. So it is worth checking that you are still wearing the correct size of shoe, even after your feet have stopped growing.

It's a great idea to kick off your shoes whenever you can and walk barefoot, as nature intended. Walking over irregular surfaces stimulates the reflexes of the feet. Sometimes, when wearing shoes it is difficult to stimulate the feet, so circulation and flexibility of the foot can decline with age. Sand is an excellent medium to walk over because its surface changes with each footstep, massaging the various aspects of the foot. If you don't have a sand pit or beach close on hand, walking barefoot on warm grass or carpet can be good alternatives. It also connects you to the earth element and helps you feel more grounded. If you are low on energy, avoid walking barefoot over cold or hard surfaces because this can further deplete your energy levels.

Spending a few minutes each day walking barefoot on warm surfaces or rolling your feet over a wooden foot roller will have a beneficial effect on your well-being. There are now some very good rollers available, which allow you to rub your feet up and down and stimulate the reflexes of your feet.

Spending a few minutes each day spreading out your toes will improve the flow of energy in those toes. You can buy "toe combs," which are often used when applying nail polish to the toenails. They are easy to use and help create some space between the toes. Alternatively, you can stand barefoot on a flat surface, and use your fingers to separate the toes. Another useful exercise to help strengthen the foot's structure and stretch calf muscles shortened by prolonged use of high-heeled shoes is to place the balls of your feet on a hardback book or piece of wood that is about 1¼ inches (3 cm high), and then place the heels of your foot on the floor.

Hands

The hands are usually open to the elements and are not restrained by ill-fitting garments, but they can get dry and rough. Using a hand cream daily will combat this and keep your skin and nails soft and supple.

Here is a further exercise, which will add flexibility and strength in the hands and fingers. Hold a small rubber ball in one hand—a yellow spot squash ball is perfect for the job. Repeatedly squeeze and then relax each one of your fingers around the ball. Repeat with your other hand. Then place two balls of a similar size in one hand—you can use squash balls or "worry balls"—and use your fingers to move the balls around so one is at the top of your hand just below the fingers and one by your wrist. Repeat the process so the balls change position, and carry on for a few minutes. Then repeat using the other hand.

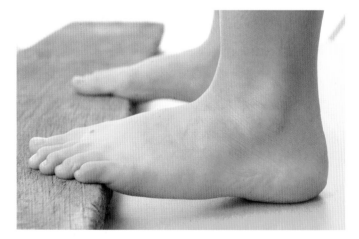

Achilles' tendon flexibility can help prevent injury. An effective way to stretch the tendon is to stand on a plank of wood. Hold for 30 seconds but do not bounce. You should feel a gentle stretch in your calf muscles.

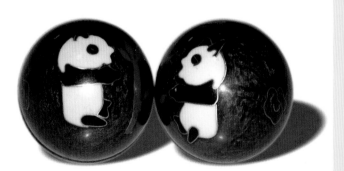

Worry balls are usually heavy and often have intricate designs. A good basic exercise is to move both balls around in one hand. Alternatively, as a massage tool, press the palms of the hands or the arches of the feet into them.

getting started

Reflexology can be used as both self-help and as a treatment for your family and friends, but whichever you choose, it is important to stick to a few basic guidelines.

Before treating someone, make sure that your nails are trimmed and your hands clean.

Before you start

Before you start any treatment it is important to ask some simple questions. Try to find out how your friends or family members want to feel at the end of the treatment. Ask them how they would benefit from feeling different, why they are feeling the way they are, and what effect their diet, lifestyle, or exercise regime have on them. This will give you important insights and help you personalize the treatment. If you want to treat yourself, you should still go through the same list of questions.

Make sure that it is safe for you or the person you are treating to receive reflexology. If you are at all unsure, check with a doctor first. It is strongly recommended that you consult your doctor if any of the following apply:

• Conditions such as diabetes, phlebitis, or thrombosis
• Suspected illness
• On medication
• Had an operation
• Any recurrent or undiagnosed pain
• Undiagnosed swelling or inflammation
• Pregnant or had a miscarriage.

Self-help

Spending a few minutes each day using the reflexes on the hands to give an uplifting and pleasurable treatment is something that you can easily do for yourself. It will help you relax more, detoxify your body, and help you feel more content, plus it will increase your energy and vitality levels.

Giving a hand reflexology treatment is often more convenient because it can be done anywhere and at any time. The hands are smaller, so the treatment is often quicker; but the hands are not as sensitive as the feet, so more treatments may be needed.

You cannot harm yourself by carrying out a self-treatment. When treating yourself it is best not to spend too much time concentrating on a single area (five to ten minutes is sufficient) because this can overstimulate the organs associated with that reflex and lead to the energies being unbalanced.

Preparing to give a treatment

Before you start giving a reflexology treatment, take time to prepare the environment.

• Ensure you have short fingernails. The optimal length is when the fingertips are visible as you look at the top of your hands.
• Consider introducing some soft lighting and soothing music.
• Ensure that the room is heated to a comfortable temperature.

• Check that the couch or chair used by the receiver is comfortable. The lower legs should be supported and possibly raised, with the feet in a relaxed position. A few pillows or throws are handy for providing cushioning on which the hand or foot can rest while you work.

• Remove shoes and socks. Any tight-fitting garments should be loosened to allow the energy to flow through the body.

Giving a treatment

The individual you are working with should have clean feet. It is best to ask the person to soak them in a footbath prior to the session or while you are getting ready. Alternatively, the feet can simply be cleaned with antiseptic wipes.

All feet are different, and a lot of useful information can be picked up by looking at the feet, especially their color, and by checking their temperature. Cold feet that look blue or red indicate poor circulation, as does dry skin on the foot. Feet that perspire may indicate a glandular imbalance.

Cracks in the soles, calluses, corns, bunions, and so on should be noted, together with the area in which they occur—for example, cracks on the heel usually indicate pelvic disorders. Also, consider which zones on the feet these features occur in, and make connections to the relevant body zone. An in-growing toenail may relate to headaches or migraine; flat feet may indicate a problem with the spine.

Feet that feel tense will inform you that the person is stressed. Limp feet tend to indicate poor muscle tone. If there is puffiness around the ankle, internal problems may be present.

Tips and advice for giving treatments and self-help

• Always start and end the treatment with a few minutes of the relaxation routines given in this book.

• Keep an eye on your posture. Try to keep your back straight and supported to help with your own flow of internal energies and to avoid backaches. Sit with the individual's face in your view, so that you can gauge his or her reaction.

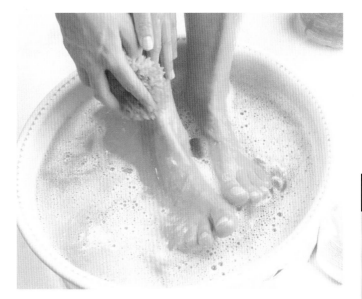

A long soak in a footbath will clean the feet and soften any hard skin, making massage easier.

• Use gentle pressure if you are working on someone who is menstruating, has osteoporosis, or is elderly or very young (under the age of 11).

• Provide a glass of water at room temperature following a treatment.

• Don't work over varicose veins, cuts, bruises, scar tissue, or damaged areas.

• Don't work over athlete's foot—this can spread the infection.

• Don't give reflexology to people with diabetes, thrombosis, or phlebitis, or to yourself if you have these conditions.

• Consult your doctor if you have any concerns following a reflexology treatment.

warning

Check that the individual you are working with does not have an extensive fungal infection, because it can easily pass to your hands. Do not work on areas where verrucas or warts exist, unless you cover them with a bandage, because these can spread to other areas of the foot, or be passed on to you.

the massage techniques

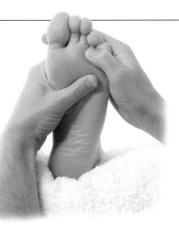

This shows the usual position of the thumb in reflexology; it is bent at an angle and pressure is applied to the pad while the holding hand supports the foot.

There are various techniques that you need to master to enable you to carry out a reflexology treatment, most of which are performed with the thumb but some with the fingers as well.

T he main technique used in reflexology treatments is the caterpillar walk (see opposite page). Other commonly applied techniques are rotating on a point, which is where you pinpoint a reflex area with the middle finger of one hand and then rotate the ankle or wrist. The hook-and-back-up technique is used for a specific point and involves exerting pressure with the thumb then "hooking in" and pulling back. Twisting, tapping, traction, applying pressure, and rolling are also used in reflexology treatments.

Each reflex is about the size of a pinhead so, for the treatment to be effective, real precision is required. The pressure applied should be firm, but not too aggressive. You want to apply pressure that is within the person's comfort zone. The hands and fingers are also used to either support the foot or provide leverage.

Some people may feel many sensations while being treated, while others will report feeling almost nothing at all. On the first session, the person may feel little or no tenderness on the foot. This does not mean that there are no areas of congestion; usually it indicates a blockage in the feet that needs to be freed. Frequently, the feet become more sensitive during subsequent sessions. The tenderness that is felt in the points representing the congested areas will also diminish over the course of treatment.

Although some pain may be felt on some of the reflexes, the treatment as a whole should not be painful. It should leave the person relaxed and refreshed.

Before (and often after) the treatment, it is important to use some relaxation techniques for the foot. These are described in more detail on pages 40–41. They have the effect of stimulating circulation, which warms the person's feet and sometimes his or her whole body. It also allows the individual to become accustomed to your touch. You may choose to relax both feet, and then begin the main treatment; or the right foot can be relaxed first and then worked on immediately, followed by the same sequence for the left foot.

KEY TO TECHNIQUE SYMBOLS

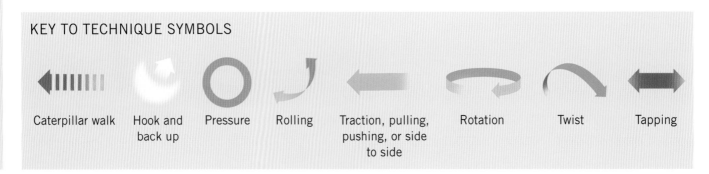

| Caterpillar walk | Hook and back up | Pressure | Rolling | Traction, pulling, pushing, or side to side | Rotation | Twist | Tapping |

Caterpillar walk

This reflexology massage technique is performed with the thumbs and fingers of both hands. As with any skill, it takes a little time and practice to master the technique; it may also take some time to build up the necessary strength. It's a good idea to practice on your forearm or hand.

How much pressure you apply is largely intuitive. It should be firm enough for the person to feel a reaction in the reflex points but not so aggressive that it causes pain. Remember that your fingers and thumb may easily tire while you're learning because they are unaccustomed to working in this way. Take regular breaks, change hands, and apply some of the hand relaxation techniques from pages 52–55. It is also useful to spend a few minutes each day strengthening the hand and digits by the exercises given for the hands on pages 34–35.

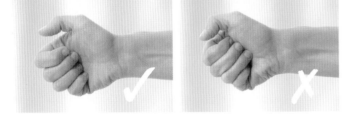

1 Angle of the thumb

The thumb is bent at about 45 degrees and "walks" along the foot or hand in very small "steps" of a fraction of an inch at a time to create a feeling of constant pressure on the surface. The forward-creeping motion is similar to how a caterpillar moves, which is why it is often called the caterpillar walk (CW). Repeat the exercise using your index finger, bending just the first joint at about 45 degrees. Do not move the first thumb joint too much, it should hardly move from one tiny step to the next.

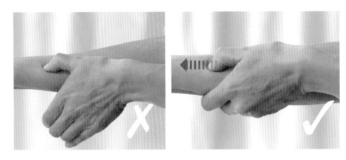

2 Applying leverage

The power the thumb or index finger has to stimulate the reflexes is increased with leverage, which can be attained by simply wrapping the hand or fingers around the foot or hand to support them. A simple experiment that demonstrates leverage is to CW up your arm with the thumb, without allowing your fingers to touch the arm. Note the pressure of the touch. Repeat the exercise, this time wrapping your fingers around your arm, and you should see that your thumb can exert a lot more pressure.

3 Applying the technique

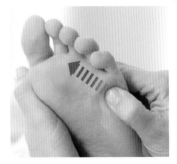

Now practice applying the technique on a foot. With the holding hand, stretch the sole of the foot to create a smooth, even surface for your thumb or finger to work. This can be achieved by resting your thumb on the sole and wrapping your fingers around the side of the foot. With your working hand, drop your wrist to create leverage. Bend and unbend the thumb's first joint, moving it forward in little steps at a time—each time you lift the thumb, move forward and apply pressure. When your hand feels stretched, reposition it and carry on "walking" it forward.

relaxing the feet

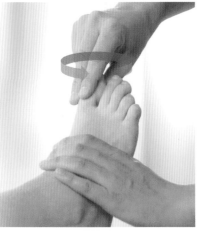

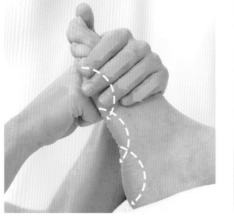

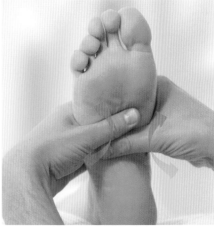

1 Toe rotation

Starting with the big toe, hold each toe with the finger and thumb of one hand, while the other hand holds the foot itself. Gently rotate the toe in one direction three times, then rotate it in the opposite direction three times. Give a gentle tug. Then repeat for the other toes, working toward the little toe in sequence.

2 Metatarsal kneading

With one hand holding the foot at the toes, clench the other hand to form a fist. Starting at the fleshy part of the sole just under the toes, use your fist to push against the foot in a kneading motion down the foot to the heel, moving the other hand down at the same time to maintain support of the person's foot. This can be repeated a few times.

3 Thumb rolling

Hold the foot by placing both sets of fingers over the front of the foot with the thumbs on the sole, one above the other, at the bottom of the heel. Then firmly and smoothly place the bottom thumb above the other one. Continue this process until the whole area from the heel to the base of the toes has been thumb rolled.

4 Spinal twist

Place the fingers of both hands side by side, holding the top of the foot by the ankle with the thumbs on the sole, in a position similar to that used when a Chinese burn is given to the wrist. The hand close to the heel is kept still, while the other hand slowly and smoothly rotates the foot back and forth. Ensure that the foot is rotated evenly in both directions. Repeat this a few times and then edge forward toward the toes, using the same technique. Continue until you reach the toes.

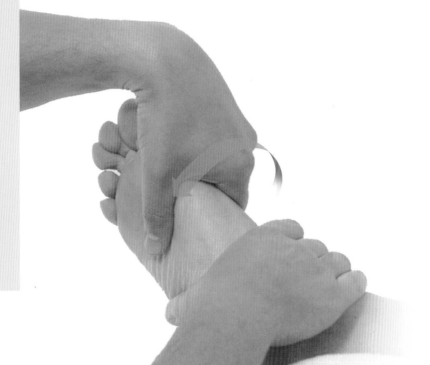

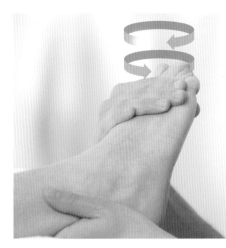

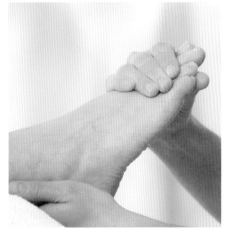

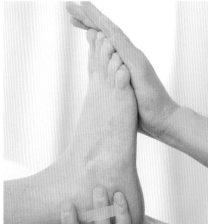

5 **Ankle rotation**

Cup the heel in one hand, and with the other hand firmly hold the toes and part of the sole. Keeping your cupped hand still, gently rotate the foot clockwise in complete circles a few times, then counterclockwise. This technique, as well as being relaxing, also stimulates the reflex that relates to the uterus and the prostate, and the whole of the hip area.

6 **Achilles' tendon stretch**

Cup the heel in one hand, and with the other hand grasp the top of the foot near the toes. Pull the toes toward you, allowing the heel to move backward, then pull the heel toward you, allowing the toes to move backward. Repeat this a few times.

Be careful to do this movement smoothly to avoid damaging the person's Achilles' tendon.

7 **Foot wobbling**

Place one palm on each side of the ankle, at right angles to the foot. Keeping the hands and wrists relaxed, rock the foot side to side by gently moving your hands back and forth in opposite directions. Gradually move the hands up from the ankle to the toes so the whole of the foot is worked on. This technique is good for relaxing the foot and lower leg, and it also aids circulation.

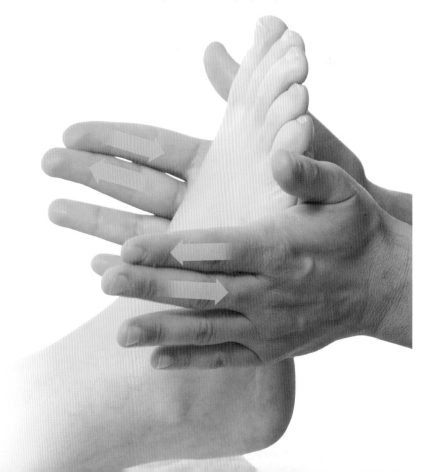

the main treatment: feet

Once the feet have been thoroughly relaxed and the person is feeling at ease, you will be ready to begin giving the main treatment.

I t is worth asking the person how he or she feels and what sensations are experienced during a treatment. These can be emotional as well as physical. Make sure that the pressure you use is comfortable for the individual, not too hard or too soft. Check three or four times during a treatment. Sometimes he or she will tell you anyway, in which case there is no need to ask! If the person falls asleep, which is common during a treatment, don't wake him or her up to ask.

When someone tells you an area is tender, release the pressure slightly and rework the area. Also, rework the area whenever you feel any blockages. Such blockages may feel like sand under the skin, or like a miniature bubble, a little like those found on bubble wrap. Keep a note for your records, so that you can compare the state of the reflex the next time a treatment is carried out.

The treatment should not be ticklish because the massage technique used should be too firm to tickle. If the person being treated finds it ticklish, increase the pressure of your stroke (but be careful not to be too firm—some reflex points can be tender).

Use a relaxing foot moisturizer or balm—peppermint is particularly good—to soften the feet because this will make it easier to work over the feet. However, don't use too much moisturizer and avoid massage oils because it is hard to contact the reflexes properly on slippery skin. Many reflexologists now prefer to use specialized creams or foot powders for giving a reflexology treatment. Talcum powder was once popular, but it has been linked to certain health problems, including cancer.

How often?

How often you have reflexology depends on whether you are trying to treat a recurring problem or just wish to stay healthy. If you are fit and healthy, then a full foot session every month should be adequate, perhaps supplemented with occasional hand treatments. If you have an ailment, such as back pain, migraines, or insomnia, 20-minute treatments targeting those areas two to three times a week would be beneficial, together with regular hand sessions.

The opposite page provides a photographic summary of the main treatment for feet that follows on pages 44–51. Initially you will need to refer to those pages as well as consult the reflex maps on pages 26–33. Once you are familiar with the sequence, after practicing them several times, you can refer to page 43 for a useful at-a-glance workout summary.

tip
If it is slightly cool, wrap a towel around the foot you are not working on.

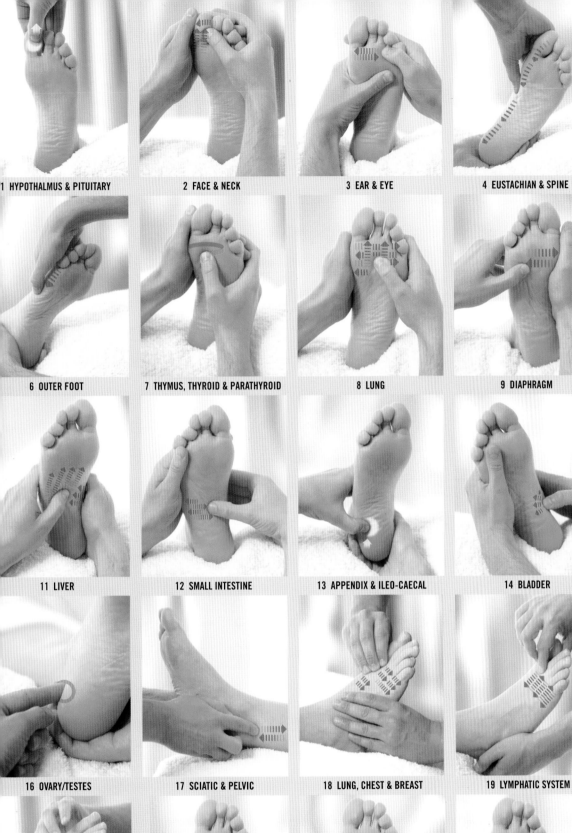

1 HYPOTHALMUS & PITUITARY
2 FACE & NECK
3 EAR & EYE
4 EUSTACHIAN & SPINE
5 SHOULDER

6 OUTER FOOT
7 THYMUS, THYROID & PARATHYROID
8 LUNG
9 DIAPHRAGM
10 SPLEEN & STOMACH

11 LIVER
12 SMALL INTESTINE
13 APPENDIX & ILEO-CAECAL
14 BLADDER
15 URETER, KIDNEY & ADRENAL

16 OVARY/TESTES
17 SCIATIC & PELVIC
18 LUNG, CHEST & BREAST
19 LYMPHATIC SYSTEM
20 GROIN

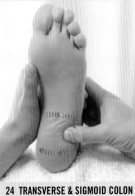
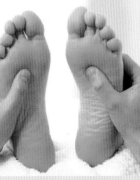

21 CIRCULATION
22 SPLEEN & STOMACH
23 SMALL INTESTINE
24 TRANSVERSE & SIGMOID COLON
25 SOLAR PLEXUS

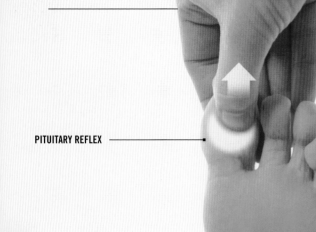

PITUITARY REFLEX

1 With the thumb in the bent position as previously described (see page 39), pinch the hypothalamus reflex by placing the hand over the toes, the fingers over the front of the toe, and the thumb over the reflex, using a pinching, squeezing motion. Repeat for the pituitary reflex.

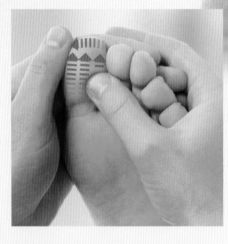

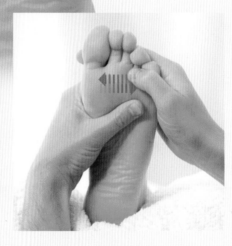

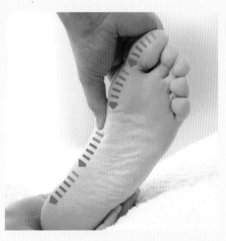

2 Caterpillar walk (CW) over the toes starting with the sole of the big toe, walking upward, then across the face reflex. With the other toes, go up the back and down the front, working toward the little toe in sequence. CW over the top of the toes in both directions. Be sensitive to what your fingers feel; tenderness is frequently felt while working on these areas. CW over the neck reflex, from the outside of the big toe toward zone 2.

3 CW over eye and ear reflex in both directions. It helps if you pull back some of the fleshy part of the ball of the foot with one hand while working these reflexes.

4 Work over the eustachian reflex, making a pinching and circular-type motion with the thumb and index finger. Work up and down the spine reflex, using CW. When you reach the heel, slightly increase the level of pressure. Many people find parts of this reflex tender, so remember to ask how the individual is feeling, and be sensitive to any areas of congestion. It is worth working the spine reflex more than once, because tension is frequently found at some part of the spine.

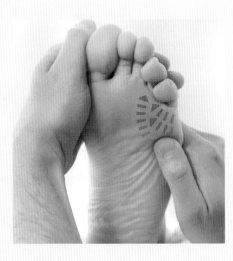

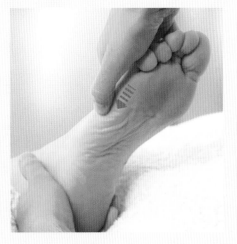

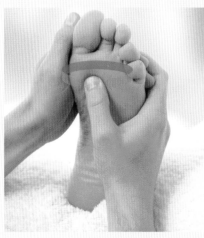

5 Work the shoulder reflex. Start low down on the sole part of the reflex, doing the CW with the thumb, working toward the toes. Then work on the shoulder reflex at the front of the foot, using the index finger to perform the CW. The shoulder reflex is often crunchy, again because of tension found in this area.

6 Work the outer foot. Starting at the bottom of the little toe, work the arm, elbow, knee, and leg reflexes, ending with the hip. Work the cuboid notch in both directions. The hip reflex should also be worked in a crisscross manner.

7 Stimulate the thymus, thyroid, and parathyroid reflexes thoroughly. The best way to do this is to make a circling motion with the thumb.

8 CW the sole part of the lung reflex, while your left hand thumbs over the diaphragm reflex, with the fingers over the front of the foot. Work this reflex both upward and in both horizontal directions. Then CW the front part of the foot from zone 5 to zone 1 over the lung reflex.

LUNG REFLEX

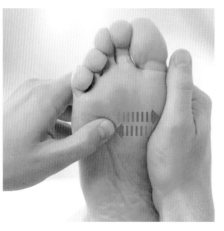

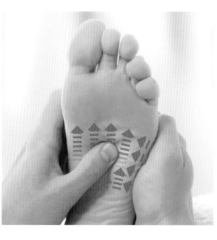

tip
It is useful to remember that the line of the diaphragm reflex also represents the dividing line between the ball and the arch of the foot.

9 CW over the line of the diaphragm reflex in both directions with your thumbs, resting your fingers on the front of the foot.

10 Work the spleen and stomach reflexes by doing the CW across zones 1 to 4.

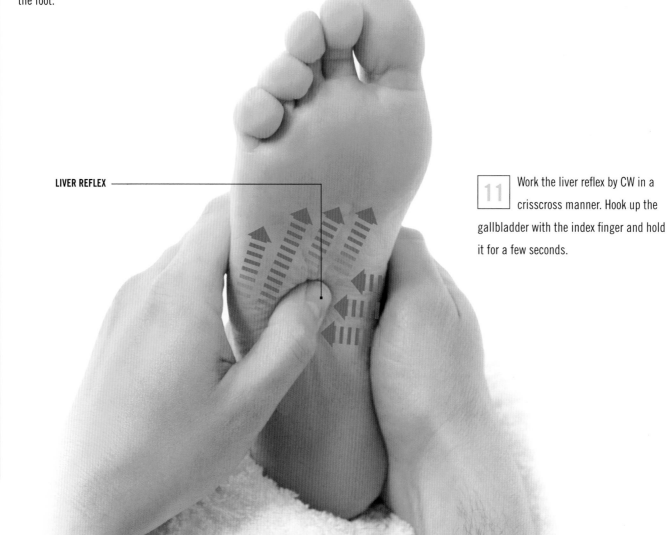

LIVER REFLEX

11 Work the liver reflex by CW in a crisscross manner. Hook up the gallbladder with the index finger and hold it for a few seconds.

SMALL INTESTINE
REFLEX

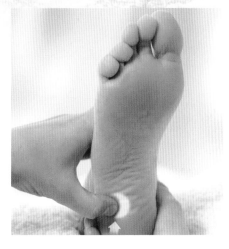

 12 Work the small intestine reflex by CW in both horizontal directions.

 13 Hook up the appendix and ileo-caecal reflex for a few seconds. CW up the ascending colon reflex and across the transverse colon reflex, ending at the instep of the right foot.

14 Work the bladder reflex by CW diagonally upward toward the little toe. The bladder, ureter, kidney, and adrenal gland reflexes can be tender, so ask the person how he or she is during this part of the treatment.

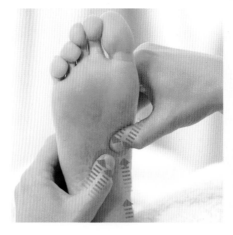

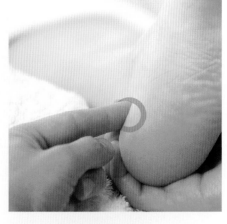

15 Work up the ureter reflex and the kidney reflex by CW, stimulate the adrenal reflex, then work down the ureter reflex and bladder reflex. Work the bladder reflex two or three times. The kidney and adrenal reflexes can be stimulated together by placing one thumb on the kidney reflex and the other on the adrenal reflex, with the two thumbs facing each other. Pull the two thumbs away from one another, and gently massage the reflexes with the thumbs for about 30 seconds.

16 Stimulate the ovary/testes reflex by circling the index finger over the reflex for a few seconds. Then, using two fingers, CW over the Fallopian tube/vas deferens reflex to the uterus/prostate reflex. Repeat the circling motion over the uterus/prostate reflex for a few seconds, and then stimulate the Fallopian tube/vas deferens reflex again, finishing at the ovary/testes reflex.

SCIATIC NERVE REFLEX

17 CW over the sciatic nerve reflex across the pelvic line near the heel and up the sides of the heel. Then, using the fingers, work up the sciatic nerve reflex on both sides of the ankle, then back down and across the pelvic line again. When doing the heel part, put more pressure on the thumbs to give a slightly harder treatment in this area.

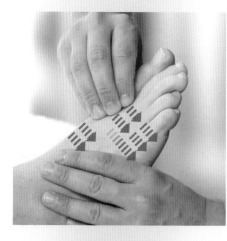 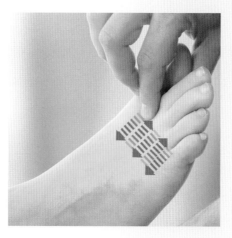

18 Using all four fingers, CW over the front of the foot starting at zone 5 and working across the foot to zone 1 to work the lung, chest, and breast reflex.

19 Massage the lymphatic system reflexes found between each toe. This is done by pinching the web between each of the toes, starting at the big toe and working toward the little toe. After you have pinched the web slowly and firmly, use both your index finger on the top of the foot and your thumb on the sole of the foot to perform a series of pinches down the metatarsals. Then come back to the web by squeezing the flesh of the foot between your finger and thumb.

LYMPH OF THE GROIN REFLEX

20 Using your fingers, gently CW around the anklebone—this is also a reflex to the lymph of the groin. Tenderness here relates to pelvic inflammation.

50

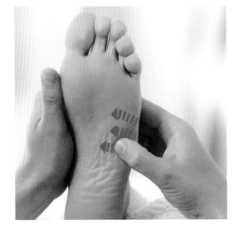

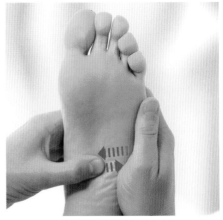

22 Work the spleen and stomach reflex by doing the CW across zones 3 to 5.

23 Work the small intestine reflex by CW in both horizontal directions.

21 Using all your fingers, gently tap (as if you were playing the piano) the whole of the front of the foot to stimulate the circulation. Now wrap a towel around the right foot and start the treatment on the left foot. Use the same massage steps as on the right foot until you finish at the diaphragm reflex.

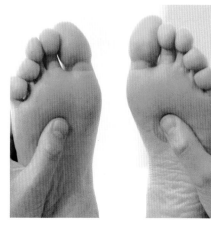

tip

Allow the person to sit quietly for some time after the treatment, particularly if he or she has been asleep; the recipient may be disorientated for a short while.

24 CW across the transverse colon reflex, down the descending colon reflex, and along the sigmoid colon, dropping just below the pelvic line at the midline, then up toward the bladder reflex. Give the rectum reflex a squeeze with the thumb.

25 Now work the rest of the left foot in a similar manner to the right foot. When both feet have had the main treatment, the solar plexus relaxation treatment can be given. This relaxation method can also be given at the start of a treatment. The solar plexus is the main storage area for stress, and applying pressure to this area can always bring about a degree of relaxation.

This technique should be applied to both feet simultaneously. Take the right foot in the left hand, and the left foot in the right hand. The fingers should be wrapped around the side of the foot, with the thumbs over the solar plexus reflex. Ask the person to inhale slowly while you press on the solar plexus reflex and exhale as you release the pressure. Do not lose contact with the foot while you are doing this. Repeat the process about three times.

SIGMOID COLON REFLEX

relaxing the hands

The following exercises will help to relax you and the person you are working on. They can provide a beginning, an end, or a transition between the techniques in the Main Treatment section.

R elaxed hands and, by extension, a relaxed person, will make your reflexology work much easier and more pleasant because the individual will be much more receptive to the techniques and routines you are about to apply.

It is equally important for you to be relaxed and to prepare your hands for the work they are about to do. Our hands are our tools, and without their flexibility and sensitivity, simple activities would become very difficult. Performing just a few minutes of these routines each day will be time well spent. In these exercises, it is best not to force any movement but instead to just let your hands ease into position.

As with the feet, these relaxation exercises will stimulate circulation and warm the person's hands, and even the whole body. It also allows him or her to get used to your touch. You may choose to relax both feet and then begin the main treatment; or the right foot can be relaxed first and then worked on immediately, followed by the same sequence for the left foot.

Before you start, remember to cut or file your fingernails so that they don't scratch or dig into the skin while you are working, and to wash your hands carefully or use antiseptic wipes. You can then apply an aqueous cream if you like.

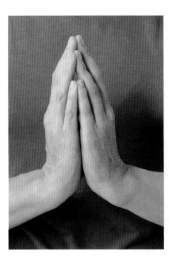

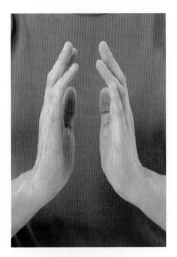

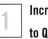 **Increasing sensitivity to Qi**

This is a useful exercise because it makes you more aware of your own Qi and also the Qi of the people you are treating. Qi is the energy that practitioners of Oriental medicine believe represents the "life force," or "life energy." Some people find this exercise easier if they close their eyes. Place your hands in a prayer position, roughly about chest height, with fingertips pointing upward.

Gradually pull your palms apart, still facing one another as before, until they are about 2 inches (5 cm) away from one another, and then slowly bring them toward each other again so that they are about ½ inch (1 cm) apart. Relax, smile, and become aware of the space between your palms. You may feel a tingling or heat, or perhaps a cold or magnetic sensation; these are all various aspects of Qi. As your sensitivity increases, you can slowly widen the gap between the palms to about 3 feet (90 cm).

2 | Thumb-and-finger rotation

This technique will loosen the joints and relax the hand. With your thumb and index finger, hold the thumb of the other hand at its bottom, on the proximal phalange (page 25). Gently move the thumb in a circular, clockwise motion, three times, and then counter-clockwise three times.

Give a gentle tug, then squeeze the thumb upward, repeating on the distal phalange (page 25). Squeeze up to the bottom of the thumbnail. Many energy meridians start or end here, and a squeeze at the bottom of the nail will help to increase the energy flow in this area.

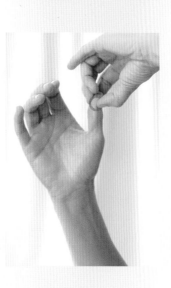

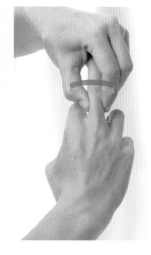

Apply more pressure at the bottom of the nail by giving it a good squeeze on both sides of the thumb. Continue to squeeze to the end of the thumb tip, so that a kind of a "snap" is produced. Be careful not to over-apply pressure by squeezing the joints of the fingers more than they can comfortably absorb.

Repeat the thumb routine on the other fingers—however, because each finger has three joints (there are only two joints in the thumb), repeat the rotations and squeezes three times, not forgetting to squeeze each side of the nail bottom. If you are working on a friend, support his or her wrist for more relaxation.

54

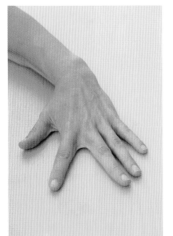

3 Palm stretching

Place one hand palm down on a table. With your index and middle finger of the other hand, make a "V" shape. Remember not to force any of the fingers into this exercise—with practice, their flexibility will improve.

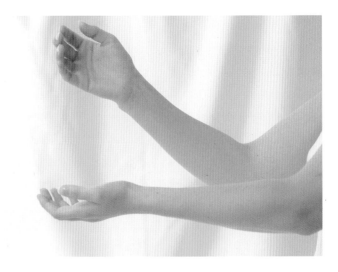

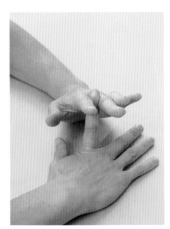

Using the "V" shape made by the one hand, lever the index finger of the other hand away from the palm so that the finger is helped to stand vertically or at a greater than 90 degree angle.

4 Hand chopping technique

This technique aims to improve hand circulation and loosen the wrists of either the person giving, or the person receiving, reflexology. It is crucial that the chopping hand is relaxed and not tense, and that the wrist is loose, almost floppy.

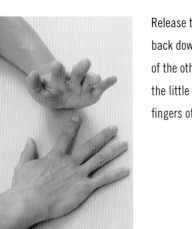

Release the index finger to "flip" back down on the table. Do each of the other fingers, finishing with the little finger. Repeat with the fingers of the other hand.

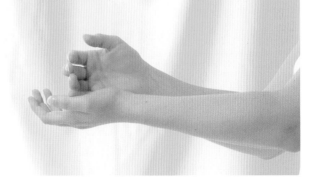

Hold out one hand, palm outstretched. If giving this to a friend, it is a good idea to support their upward palm in your palm for added comfort. Use the sides of your hands in a chopping motion (without the tension) to lightly slap the palm of the outstretched hand. Repeat on both hands.

5 Wrist exercises

Hold your hand or your friend's hand by wrapping your fingers around the top of his or her relaxed hand. Breathe in. Pull the hand gently and smoothly away from the wrist joint as the breath is exhaled. Let go and repeat twice, and then repeat the technique on the other hand.

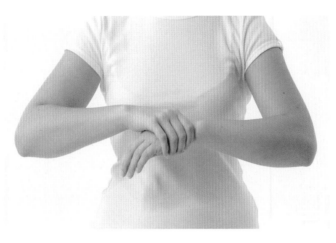

Keeping both wrists relaxed and loose, shake both hands at the same time, like drops of water spraying a wet cloth. Imagine all the debris and negative energy leaving your hands and wrists.

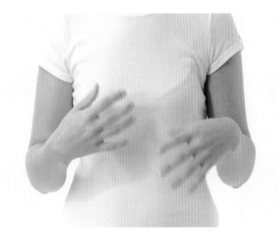

With your hands at heart level close to your chest and your elbows spread (see page 52), slowly move both hands down toward your waist until you feel the heel of the hands beginning to pull apart. This exercise will improve wrist flexibility.

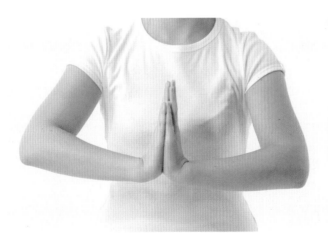

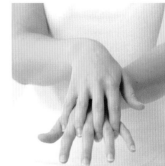

6 Stroking

Place one hand palm facing downward. Then, place the other hand so that each finger touches the web of the opposite hand's finger.

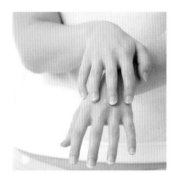

Now gently stroke the back of the first hand by drawing the upper hand toward the wrist of the bottom hand. Repeat this action two more times and then move to the other hand. Be sure to stroke only in one direction.

the main treatment: hands

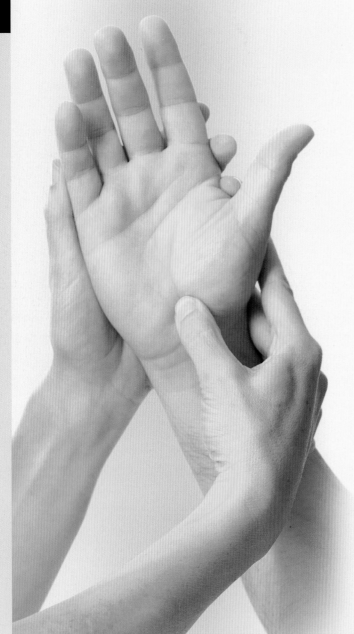

With the hands and wrists now completely relaxed, you should be ready to begin the main hand reflexology treatment.

T reating yourself or others using hand reflexology has the same effects as using the feet, but it has the advantage of being more convenient, because it can be carried out in any place, at any time, such as on the train to work, in your lunch break, or even in the bath. Although ideally it would be good to get the external environment correct, such as the lighting and surrounding ambience, it is not essential.

The main difference between the hands and the feet is that the areas are more condensed in the hands. The hands are also more exposed to the elements and not as sensitive as the feet. Generally, this will mean that more treatments will be required for hand reflexology than for foot reflexology.

The opposite page provides a photograph summary of the main treatment for hands that follows on pages 58–63. Initially you will need to refer to those pages as well as consult the reflex maps on pages 30–33. Once you have practiced a few times, you can refer to the opposite page for a useful at-a-glance summary of the reflexes.

Like the feet, particular places on the hands reflect certain areas of the body. Once the basic layout has been learned, finding the reflexes is easy.

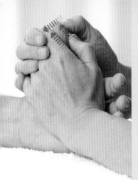

1 HEAD

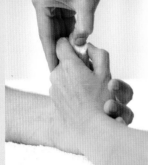

2 PITUITARY

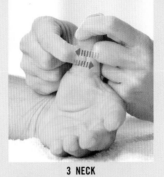

3 NECK

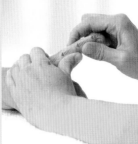

4 SINUS

5 EUSTACHIAN TUBE

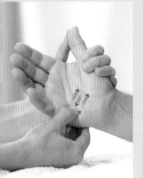

6 SPINE

7 SHOULDER

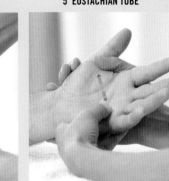

8 KNEE/LEG/HIP/LOWER BACK

9 LUNG

10 DIAPHRAGM

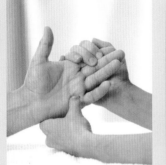

11 LIVER & GALLBLADDER

12 STOMACH (ZONE 1)

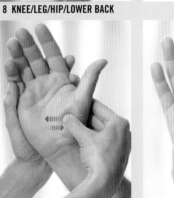

13 SMALL INTESTINE

14 LARGE INTESTINE

15 TRANSVERSE COLON

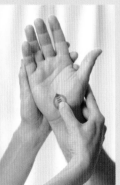

16 BLADDER

17 KIDNEY & ADRENAL

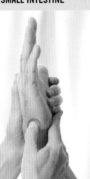

18 OVARY/TESTES

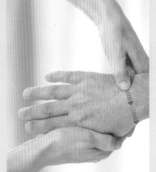

19 FALLOPIAN TUBE/VAS DEFERENS

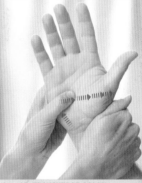

20 LUNG

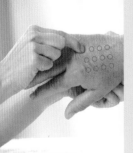

21 LYMPHATIC SYSTEM

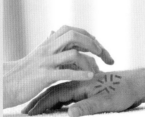

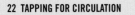

22 TAPPING FOR CIRCULATION

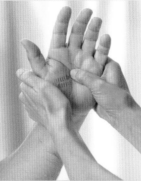

23 STOMACH & SPLEEN

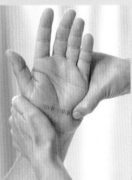

24 DESCENDING COLON

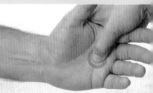

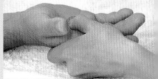

25 SOLAR PLEXUS

58

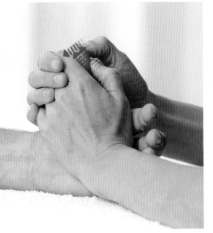

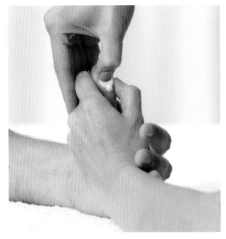

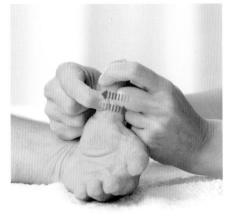

1 With the right hand, caterpillar walk (CW) around the outside of the thumb. Start just above the outside edge of the thumb joint, moving over the top of the thumb and down the other side to the web between the thumb and index finger. CW up the back of the top joint of the thumb, covering the whole area of the fleshy part of the thumb (this represents the head reflex) and then across the front of the thumb below the nail (the face reflex).

2 Using a pinching-and-squeezing motion similar to that used for the big toe, pinch the pituitary reflex, found roughly in the middle of the fleshy part of the thumb. Repeat with the hypothalamus, which is just above the pituitary reflex.

3 Using the CW technique, work across the back of the bottom joint of the thumb (the neck reflex). The neck reflex can be worked in both horizontal directions. There is often congestion here, so a few seconds will be well spent working this area.

4 In a similar way, work each of the fingers, starting with the index finger and finishing with the little finger. However, with the front of the fingers, work down each finger toward the hand. The palm side of the four fingers represents the sinus reflexes, and the teeth reflexes are found on the front part of the fingers. The pituitary and hypothalamus reflex is only found on the thumbs and big toes, so the fingers do not need to be "pinched."

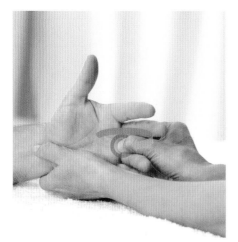

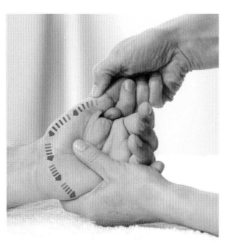

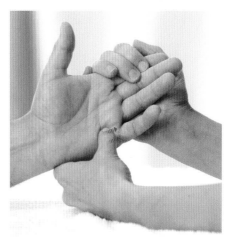

5 CW over the bottom of the index and middle fingers (eye reflex) and the base of the fourth and little fingers (ear reflex), in both directions. Work the eustachian reflex by pinching the web between the third and fourth fingers, and rotating this with the thumb and index finger.

6 Work down the spine reflex. This starts on the outside edge of the thumb just below the thumbnail, travels along the outside edge of the hand across the wrist crease, and ends at the small bone under the little finger on the wrist crease. The spine reflex on the hand is not as sensitive as that of the foot, so you can use firmer pressure here. Note any tender areas, because this will inform you of any congestion of the spine. It is worth working this reflex more than once, because we often store tension in the neck, shoulders, and at the bottom of the spine.

7 CW over the shoulder reflex. Start just below the joint at the bottom of the little finger and trace down, using the CW technique to the web between the little finger and the fourth finger. Fill the area, then work toward the other fingers. This reflex often feels "crunchy," due to tension in the shoulders. Now work the front of the shoulder reflex—this is found in roughly the same position as on the palm side, but on the top of the hand.

8 Work the outer side of the hand. Starting just below the little finger, CW down the arm, elbow, knee, and finally to the hip, leg, and lower back reflexes. These are all found on the outer edge of the little finger side of the hand. The knee, hip, leg, and lower back reflexes, which are found on the top of the hand in front of the wrist bones, should be worked in a crisscross manner.

60

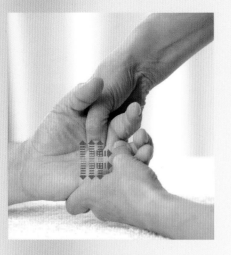

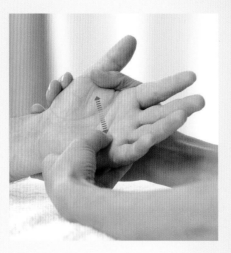

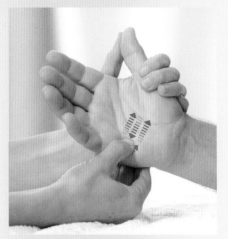

9 Crossing all four zones, the lung reflex is found under the fingers on both the palm side and on the back of both hands. CW across this lung reflex in both directions and also upward from the diaphragm reflex. Then, as in the foot, CW over the front part of the hand, over the lung reflex from the little finger side toward the thumb.

10 Work the diaphragm reflex in both directions. This is found where the phalanges meet the metacarpals, across the five zones on both the hands.

11 The liver reflex is found in the palm of the right hand. As in the foot, it is between the diaphragm and waistline, filling up most of this area and the area between zones 3 and 5. CW this reflex in a crisscross manner, and hook up to the gallbladder reflex, found in zone 4, roughly in the middle of the liver reflex.

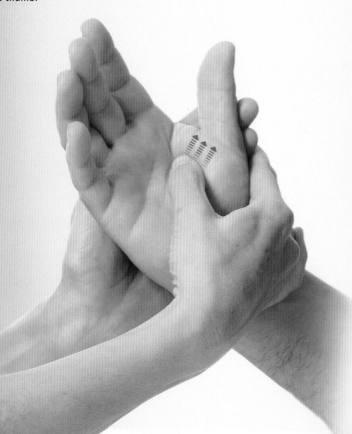

12 CW over the stomach reflex, on the right hand in zone 1, between the diaphragm reflex and the waistline.

61

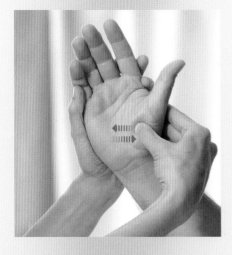 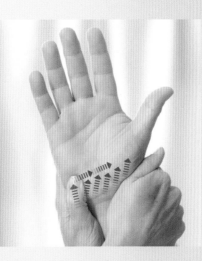 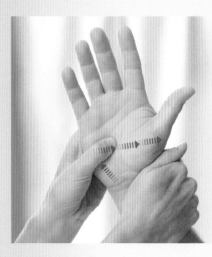

13 CW the small intestine reflex in both directions, horizontally. This reflex is found in both palms, in between the waistline and just above the wrist from zones 1 to 4.

14 The large intestine reflex area is found on the palms of both hands. It takes a similar pathway to that of the feet, starting on the right palm at the ileo-caecal valve reflex, and going up the ascending colon. It then turns at a right angle just below the waistline to become the transverse colon reflex and goes across the palm of the hand, extending to the left palm, and crossing all five zones. At the splenic flexure, between zones 4 and 5, it takes another right angle and bends down into the descending colon.

15 A short distance above the wrist, another right-angle turn is made into the sigmoid reflex, which extends across the palm above the wrist and ends in the rectum reflex, just under the middle finger, by the bladder reflex. Work this section by hooking up the appendix and ileo-caecal reflex for a few seconds. CW up the ascending colon and across the transverse colon, ending on the thumb side of the right hand.

16 CW the bladder reflex, just above the wrist crease under the middle finger, by moving upward from the wrist crease toward the fingers. Next, work up to the ureter, bladder, and adrenal gland reflexes—gently massaging the latter reflex by forming small circles slightly higher and to the thumb side of the kidney reflex will stimulate it.

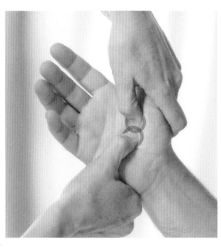

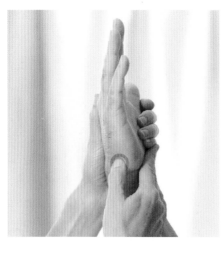

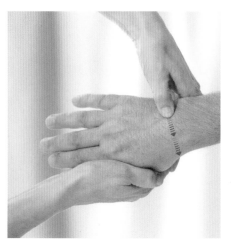

17 The kidney reflex is found in both palms under the index finger, a third of the way up the palm from the wrist crease. The ureter reflex links the bladder and kidney reflex.

18 Stimulate the ovary/testes reflex, which is found on the little finger side of the wrist crease just in front of a small wrist bone, by circling the thumb over the reflex for a few seconds.

19 CW over the top of the hand at the wrist (the Fallopian tube/vas deferens reflex) to the uterus/prostate reflex, on the thumb side of the edge of the hand, near the tendon. Stimulate this reflex as per the ovary/testes reflex.

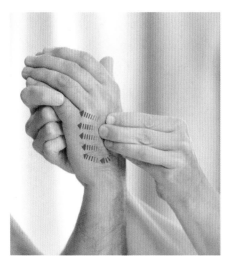

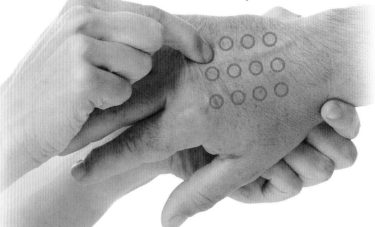

20 Using all four fingers, CW over the top of the hand, starting in zone 5 and ending at zone 1, to stimulate the lung reflex.

21 Starting at the thumb and ending with the little finger, massage the lymphatic system reflexes by pinching the web between each finger and, using your index finger and thumb, perform a series of pinches down the hand to about halfway down the palm. Return to each finger web, squeezing the flesh of the palm between your finger and thumb as you go.

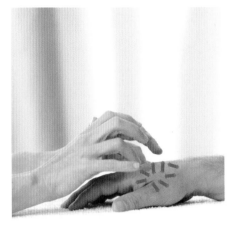

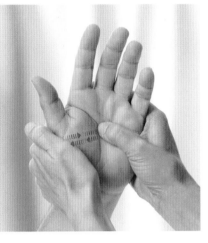

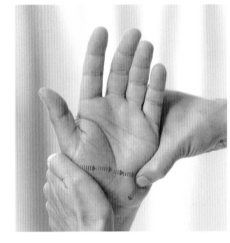

22 Using all your fingers, gently tap the top of the hand to stimulate the circulation in the hand.

Now repeat the same sequence in the left hand until you finish the diaphragm reflex.

23 CW across zones 1 to 4 to work the stomach and spleen reflex between the diaphragm and waistline. Work the small intestine reflex as before.

24 CW across the transverse colon reflex in the left hand, down the descending colon and just above the wrist crease to about halfway, under the middle finger.

Then work the left hand in a similar way to the rest of the right hand.

25 The solar plexus reflex can now be worked on both palms. As in the feet, it is worth spending a little time—20 seconds or so—on this reflex, which is found just below the diaphragm reflex, under the second and third fingers of both palms. Apply this technique in a similar manner to the feet. Gently press the solar plexus reflex as you, or the person you are working on, breathes in and release the pressure as the breath is exhaled. Repeat three times. Finish off the treatment with a couple of relaxation routines, taking a few moments before you, or the recipient, get up to be fully present in your surroundings.

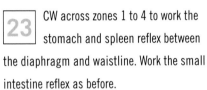

treating specific conditions

There are many conditions that respond particularly well to reflexology, such as travel sickness and earache. However, some disorders are not suitable, and people may experience a range of reactions after treatment.

T reatments for specific ailments, such as headaches, can be carried out for your friends or family, or you can treat yourself for certain problems, such as lack of energy and vitality. These are covered in more detail in the next few pages. You cannot harm yourself by carrying out self-treatment. However, be careful to avoid overstimulating one area, because this may lead to your energies being unbalanced.

Number of treatments required

Every person is different, so it is not possible to predict the exact number of sessions that will be required. Most forms of disease will have been building up over a period of time. It is, therefore, unrealistic to expect an instantaneous improvement. Serious diseases usually take longer to treat than minor ones. Likewise, disorders that have been present for a long time often require more treatments than those that have been present for only a short time. Older people may also be slower than younger people to respond to treatment.

For all diseases, a course of treatment is advised, even if the symptoms ease off after the first treatment. For the majority of disorders, six to eight weekly sessions is recommended. Usually some kind of improvement will occur after about three sessions. If, after four sessions, there does not seem to be any noticeable change to the person, then perhaps reflexology is not the best path for him or her.

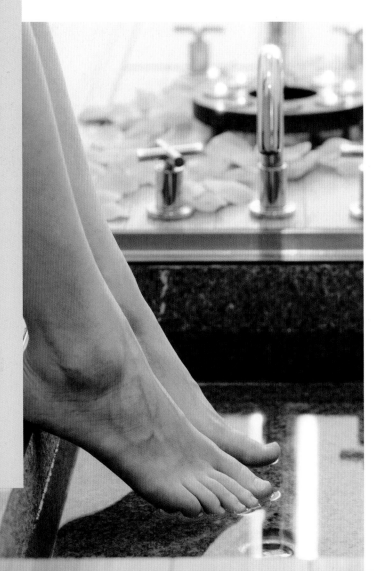

There are few people who do not benefit in some way from reflexology.

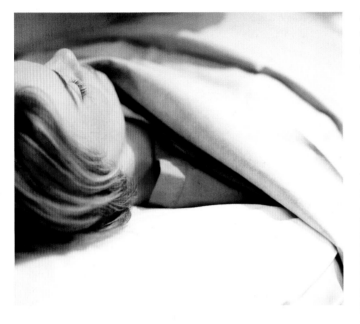

Ask the person how he or she is feeling after the treatment has finished. Have a blanket or some warm towels on hand in case the person is feeling cold.

Reactions to treatments

In order for the body to heal itself, it has to remove toxic substances that can lead to a healing crisis. The severity of the healing crisis depends upon the person. To prevent the person from having too strong a healing crisis, it is best to give a gentle first treatment. Once the treatment has finished, the person should feel relaxed and perhaps warmer, because of the stimulation of the blood circulation. Sometimes, however, the person may feel cold—this is from the toxins leaving the body.

Some of the more common reactions that may occur include:

- The person will have a very good night's sleep.
- The rate of urination may increase. The color and smell of the urine may also change.
- The person may get a cold.
- Some people experience a headache. If this does occur, it is best not to take any medication to try to suppress it.
- Suppressed past conditions could flare up.

These are all positive reactions, and show that the body is trying to heal itself. The healing crisis is usually short-lived, leaving the person with a heightened feeling of well-being.

Precautions

As previously stated, most disorders will benefit from a reflexology treatment. There are some conditions, however, for which reflexology is unsuitable. These include the following:

- Conditions requiring surgery
- Lymphatic cancer
- Early pregnancy (under 16 weeks), or pregnancies where the woman has a history of miscarriage
- Some of the more serious circulatory problems, such as phlebitis
- Deep-vein thrombosis
- Serious cases of fungal or viral foot infections, such as athlete's foot (in this case, a reflexology treatment can be done on the hands).

The following conditions can be treated with reflexology, but make sure you are careful. If you are unsure about treating any of the following disorders, then do not treat.

- Heart conditions. Here, be careful you don't overstimulate the heart. Usually a much gentler treatment is given.
- Epilepsy. In this case, be careful you don't overstimulate the brain, spinal cord, and eyes.
- Diabetes.

treating
stress

66

Stress levels can rise for any number of reasons, from trying to do too many things at once, to coping with a distressing personal issue.

Working the hands. This 20-minute routine works on key areas, such as the solar plexus, spine, and chest, giving you the strength and calmness to tackle whatever comes your way.

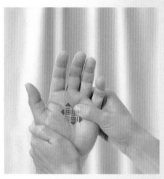

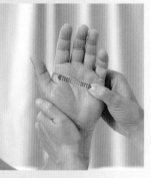

3 Work the lung reflex using the CW in all directions, to ease chest congestion.

4 Work across the diaphragm reflex in both directions to help with breathing.

5 Balance your emotions by using your thumb to gently massage the solar plexus reflex on both hands.

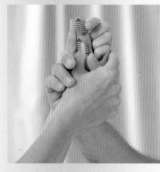

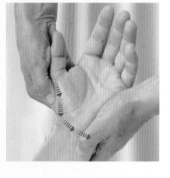

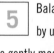

1 To help still your mind, take one finger at a time and CW around its edge, moving up its back, 2–3 times, then moving down the front, 1–2 times.

2 Relax your entire body by working down the spine reflex, starting just below the thumbnail and ending on the little finger side of the wrist crease. This also helps calm your nerves.

Working the feet. The foot tends to be more sensitive to pressure than the hand—using this 20-minute routine may help resolve more long-standing symptoms of stress.

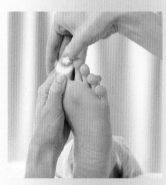 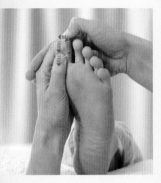 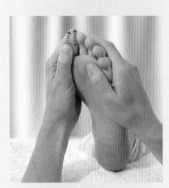 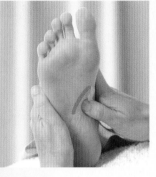

 1 Begin with a few foot relaxation techniques, such as toe rotation and the foot wobble. Then work on the big toe, pinching it between the thumb and index finger, to stimulate the pituitary reflex.

2 Continuing to work on the pituitary reflex, CW around the edge of the big toe to balance your hormones and promote a feeling of well-being.

3 CW up the back of the toe 2–3 times, then down the front of the toe, 1–2 times. Move on to the next toe. This exercise will help slow racing thoughts and reduce anxiety.

4 Work the adrenal gland reflex by forming small circles slightly higher and to the thumb side of the kidney reflex. Stimulating these glands will help produce that "feel-good" factor.

 5 Balance your emotions and allow yourself to "let go" by gently massaging the solar plexus reflex on both feet with your thumb.

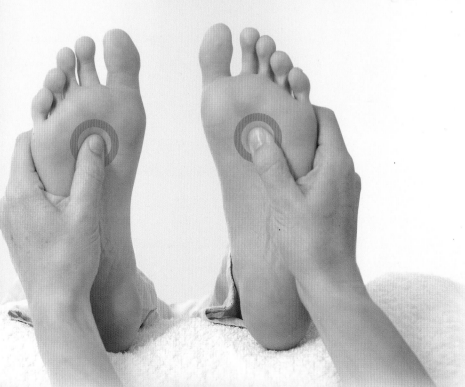

treating
headaches

68

Headaches happen for many reasons, but the main culprits are stress and hormones. To treat hormone-related headaches, which occur once or twice a month, see the PMS section; here, we look at ways to ease stress headaches.

Working the hands. This 10–15-minute routine, which focuses on the adrenal gland and head reflexes, can be repeated three times a week. For persistent headaches, consult your doctor before carrying out these self-help routines.

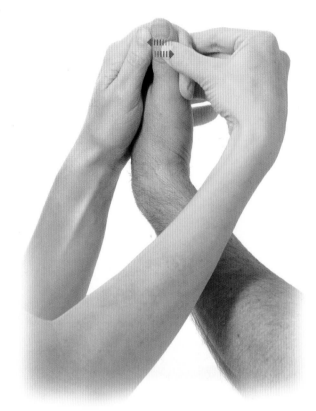

1 Work the face, head, and sinus reflexes of each of the fingers, starting with the thumb. This will ease congestion and tension.

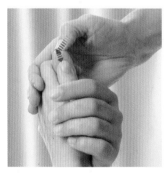

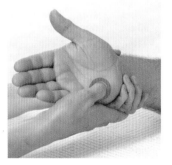

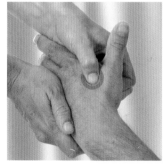

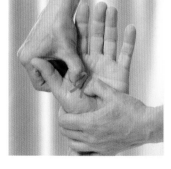

2 Focus on the brain reflex of the thumb, squeezing the fleshy part between your thumb and index finger. Move on to each of the other fingers, working the brain, face, and sinus reflexes, then work the other hand.

3 To help eliminate waste and toxins from your body, work the large intestine reflex on both hands. Spend some time working the ileo-caecal valve reflex (shown above), which is only found on the right hand.

4 A useful pressure point for headaches is found by pinching the area between your thumb and index finger, just before the two metacarpal bones meet. Hold this point, squeezing it slightly, for five or so seconds.

5 Form small circles slightly higher and to the thumb side of the kidney reflex to stimulate the adrenal glands and help control pain. Then use your thumbs to gently massage the solar plexus reflex on both hands.

Working the feet. If done regularly, this can be very beneficial for those prone to stress or tension headaches. Make sure you complete this 15-minute routine to get the most out of the treatment, and make a note of any tender areas that will indicate where more work is needed.

1 Start with some foot relaxation techniques. Then, using your thumb, hook up and squeeze the pituitary reflex to help balance your hormones.

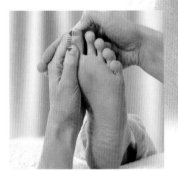

2 Taking one toe at a time, CW around the edge of the toe, up the back of it 2–3 times, and down the front 1–2 times; then move on to the next toe. This will not only help still your mind but will help to unblock the sinuses, releasing pressure in and around the head.

3 CW across the neck reflex, working the whole of the neck area. This will help to relax the neck muscles.

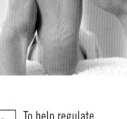
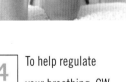

4 To help regulate your breathing, CW across the diaphragm reflex in both directions.

treating
backache

Back pain can be hard to ease, and it can range from a general pain in the upper, middle, or lower back to a specific twinge in the shoulders or neck.

If you have chronic or serious back problems, ask your doctor before you embark on these self-help techniques. This 10-minute routine can improve circulation, ease pain, and reduce tension in the spine, neck, shoulder, and lower back, keeping your muscles and joints relaxed and supple.

 1 Warm up with a few hand relaxation techniques, such as thumb rotation. Then CW across the neck reflex, working the whole of the neck area, which will help relax these muscles.

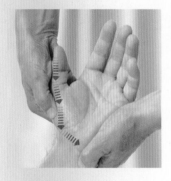

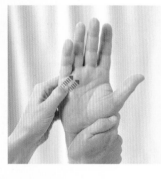

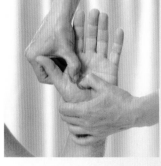

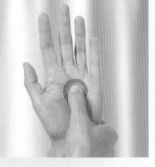

 2 Work down the spine reflex, starting just below the thumbnail and ending on the little finger side of the wrist crease to calm the body.

3 Work the whole of the shoulder reflex at the bottom of the little finger. This reflex often feels crunchy due to tension in the shoulders.

4 Work the adrenal gland reflex, found in the center of the palm. This will stimulate these glands, regulate hormones, and help with pain control.

5 Work the sacro-ileac joint, found on the wrist crease on the top of both hands, under the ring finger, to help relax the lower back. To calm the body, massage the solar plexus reflex with your thumb on both hands.

treating
constipation

Constipation occurs when a person has difficulty in opening the bowels. It may be caused by any number of things, from dietary issues, such as a lack of fiber in the diet or not drinking sufficient water, to allergies, stress, or having a general lack of vitality.

Reflexology can help release the blockages in your digestive system, allowing your body to let go of emotional issues and tension, and boost your energy levels. This 15-minute routine can be repeated up to three times a week.

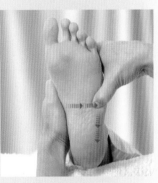 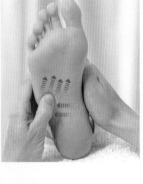

3 Working both the small and large intestine reflex will help relax this area.	**4** Work the liver reflex on the right foot to help detoxify your body.

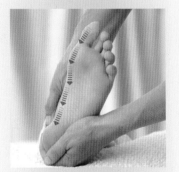 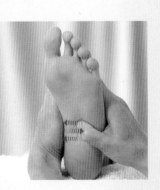

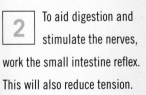

1 Start with a foot relaxation technique, such as the spinal twist. To relax the lower spine, work down the spine reflex.

2 To aid digestion and stimulate the nerves, work the small intestine reflex. This will also reduce tension.

5 Work the gallbladder reflex to aid fat digestion (as shown here), then, using your thumbs, massage the solar plexus reflex on both feet to calm the body.

treating
premenstrual syndrome
bloating and backaches

Premenstrual syndrome, or PMS, can occur between two weeks to one day before menstruation, with the symptoms often easing in the first few days of your period. Bloating and backache may be due to fluid retention, and dull or sharp cramps may occur in the pelvic area.

Working the feet. Practice this self-help routine before your period to improve your circulation, reduce cramps and bloating, and stimulate your endocrine system. It should take about 20 minutes and can be practiced up to three times a week before your period begins, and/or at the end of menstruation. It is best to take a break and not perform this routine during your period.

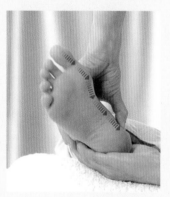

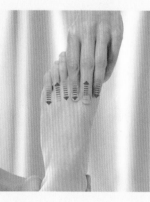

3 Work the liver reflex, which is only found in the right foot. This will help remove the toxins from your blood and improve blood flow, helping with cramps and blood clots.

1 Start with some foot relaxation techniques, then work the whole of the spine reflex to help stimulate the nerves to the various organs and relax the lower spine.

2 To reduce swelling in the breast area, massage the breast lymphatic system on the top part of the foot.

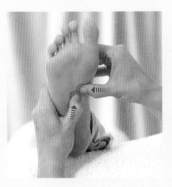

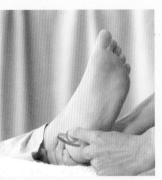

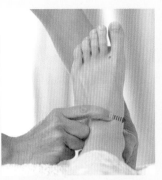

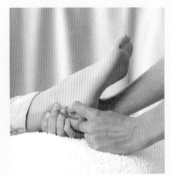

4 CW over the kidney and adrenal gland reflexes to balance water levels and maintain mineral levels. Stimulating the adrenal glands will help to control pain and balance your body's energy. In the left foot, work the spleen reflex to help detoxify your body.

5 Work the reproductive system reflexes, starting with the uterus reflex, which is located halfway between the heel and the inside anklebone. This will help increase circulation and improve blood flow.

6 Stimulating the Fallopian tube reflex, located in a horizontal band running across the top of both feet at the bottom of the ankle, will help reduce tension and "clear out" the area.

7 Working the ovaries reflex, halfway between the heel and the outside anklebone, will help produce estrogen and progesterone. Massage the solar plexus reflex to calm the body.

Working the hands. This simple routine can be performed anywhere, but it is best done up to three times a week before your period begins, and/or at the end of menstruation.

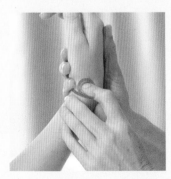

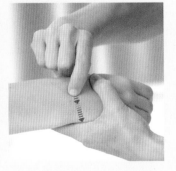

3 Work the ovaries reflex, on the outside "indent" of the wrist, to help produce and regulate estrogen and progesterone.

1 Work the uterus reflex, located on the inside of the wrist, in the indent near the wrist bone, to relax this area.

2 Stimulate the Fallopian tube reflex, located in a horizontal band running across the top of the wrist.

treating
premenstrual
syndrome

emotional and headaches

For women, hormone levels change around the time of menstruation, stirring up emotions and perhaps causing feelings of irritability and confusion, as well as headaches and migraines.

Working the hands. This routine works on the whole body to balance the endocrine system and help with mood swings and headaches. It can be practiced 2–3 times a week in the week before menstruation and takes about 20 minutes.

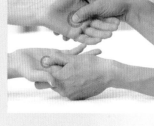

1 Start with some hand relaxation techniques. Then, using your thumb, hook up and squeeze the pituitary reflex on both thumbs. This will help balance your hormones. To help still your mind and release tension, work each one of the fingers.

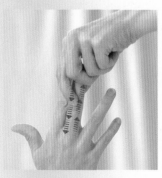

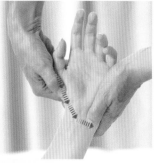

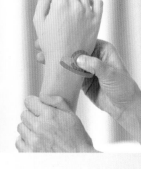

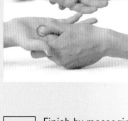

2 One finger at a time, CW around the edge of the finger, then up its back, 2–3 times, moving down the front of the finger 1–2 times. Move on to the next finger.

3 Work down the whole of the spine reflex to help relax the spine and release muscular tension.

4 To help relax the lower back, work the sacroileac joint, found on the wrist crease on the top of both hands, under the ring finger.

5 Finish by massaging the solar plexus reflex to help to balance the emotions.

Working the feet. This 20-minute routine should alleviate some of the symptoms of premenstrual syndrome by calming the body and reducing congestion in the pelvic area.

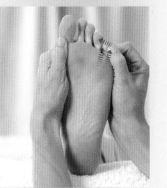

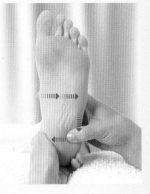

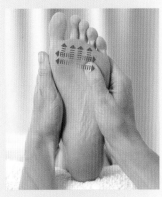

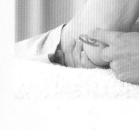

1 Still your mind and release tension by working each of the toes. One toe at a time, CW around the edge of the toe, CW up its back, 2–3 times, before working down the front 1–2 times. Move on to the next toe.

2 To "let go" and reduce bloating, work the large intestine reflex above the heel.

3 CW the whole of the lung and diaphragm reflexes. This will help to lift your spirits.

4 Work the uterus, ovaries, and Fallopian tube reflexes to ease congestion.

5 To help relax the lower back, work the sacro-ileac joint.

treating
insomnia

When you find it hard to get to sleep, or if you wake up frequently during the night, use reflexology to relax your mind, body, and spirit. Ideally, this can be carried out by someone else, so that you can lie back and fall asleep!

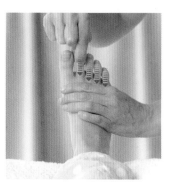

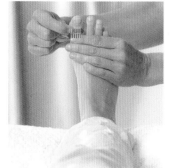

If you are working on someone else, work the feet; otherwise, the treatment may be adapted for self-treatment on the hands.

2 CW over the toes, starting with the sole of the big toe. Walk upward, then across the face reflex found on the front of the big toe. Now work on the other toes, moving up the back and down the front, working toward the little toe.

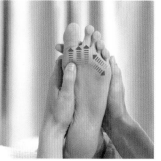

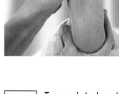

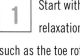

1 Start with some foot relaxation techniques, such as the toe rotation exercise, shown here, and foot wobbling.

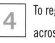

3 Work the whole of the chest reflex area, including the heart reflex, to harmonize your breathing and help relax the heart muscle.

4 To regulate breathing, CW across the diaphragm reflex in both directions. Calm the body by massaging the solar plexus reflex on both feet.

76

treating
hangovers

Feeling unwell the morning after a night of drinking alcohol is a common complaint, and you may be experiencing anything from nausea, fatigue, and a headache to dehydration or poor concentration.

Reflexology will help to remove the toxins that have entered your body, as well as balance your water levels and calm your nervous system. Practice this self-help routine for about 20 minutes at the onset of your hangover.

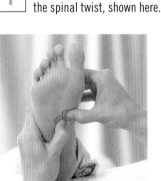

 1 Begin with a few minutes of foot relaxation techniques, such as the spinal twist, shown here.

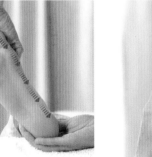

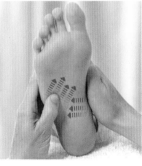

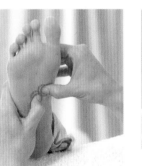

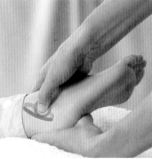

2 CW down your spine reflex to relax the spine and release any tension there while stimulating the nerves to the various organs.

3 To remove toxins from your bloodstream, CW the liver reflex, which is found toward the outer edge of the middle of the right foot.

4 Work the kidney and adrenal gland reflexes to help regulate your hormones and balance your water levels.

5 Work your sacro-ileac joint to relax the lower back. To calm the body, finish by working the solar plexus reflex.

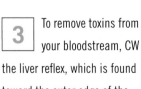

treating
panic attacks and anxiety

Anxiety can be triggered by fear, shock, or stress. It can make us feel breathless, light-headed, cold, and sweaty. When anxiety reaches extreme levels, it can lead to a panic attack, with more pronounced symptoms. By focusing on relaxing the diaphragm, reflexology can help calm the body, quickly and effectively.

It is best to practice this 5-minute routine right at the beginning of an anxiety or panic attack to help calm the breathing and bring the body back into a relaxed state.

1 Begin with a few hand relaxation techniques, then CW down the spine reflex to help relax your whole body.

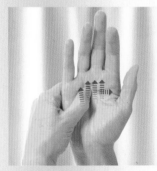 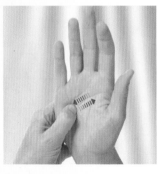

2 Work the lung reflex to regulate your breathing.

3 CW the diaphragm reflex in both directions to relax this area of the body and allow you to take deep breaths.

4 Work the adrenal gland reflex. This will balance the hormones in these glands, which are likely to be in overdrive.

5 Finish by working the solar plexus reflex, which will help to further calm you down and give a sense of well-being.

treating
hiccups

Caused by spasms of the diaphragm that create involuntary "hic" sounds at regular intervals, hiccups that refuse to subside can be a simple annoyance or source of embarrassment, but if prolonged, they can cause severe pain around the ribcage.

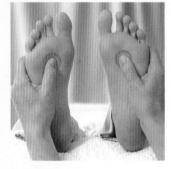

This 5-minute routine, which can be done when hiccups first start, will help calm the diaphragm.

1 Begin with a few minutes of foot relaxation techniques, such as thumb rolling, shown here.

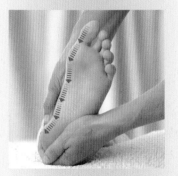

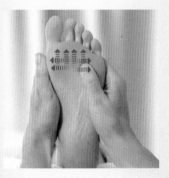

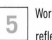

2 To help relax your whole body, CW down the spine reflex on the inside of each foot.

3 Work the entire lung reflex area to improve breathing and release tension.

4 CW the diaphragm reflex in both directions to relax this area of the body.

5 Work the solar plexus reflex for a minute or two, or until the hiccups stop.

treating
eye strain

Staring at a computer screen or focusing too intently on detailed work can cause blurred vision, headaches, a heavy feeling in the eyelids, bloodshot eyes, and even dizziness.

Working the hands. Practice this 10-minute routine at the onset of any kind of dizziness, headache, or focusing problems.

Working the feet. Practice this 10-minute routine three times a week to relieve tension around the eyes.

1 Begin with a few hand relaxation techniques, then CW up each one of the fingers, starting with the thumb and finishing with the little finger. This will help clear congestion from the sinuses and release tension in your head.

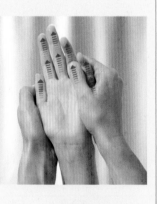

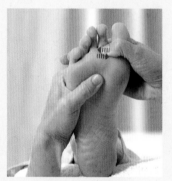

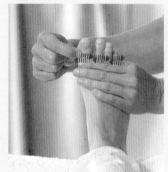

1 Work the eye reflex, which is located below the first bend of the second toe, to relax the eye muscles.

2 Work the face reflex by using your right index finger to CW along each toe. Change hands and do the same for the left foot.

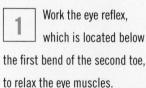

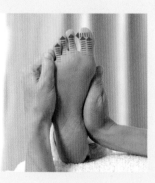

3 Work each one of the toes, starting with the big toe and finishing with the little toe. Move on to the other foot. This will clear congestion from the sinuses and release tension in your head.

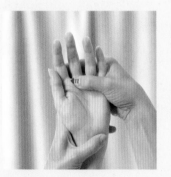

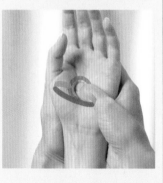

2 Work the eye reflex, between the ring and middle finger, to relax the eyes.

3 To remove toxins, CW over the kidney reflex. Work the solar plexus reflex for calmness.

treating
earache

Pain in one or both ears is often caused by the build-up of fluid in the middle ear, which can then become infected. If you have severe earaches, consult your doctor before doing any of these self-help techniques.

Working the hands. Reflexology can help prevent and alleviate earache by strengthening the immune system and releasing the build-up of toxins in the body. For the most effective results, practice this 5-minute routine 3–4 times a week, and use it in conjunction with the adjacent foot routine.

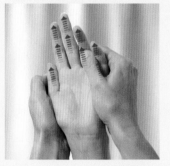

1 Work each finger, to clear sinus congestion. Move on to the kidney reflex to remove toxins, then the adrenal gland reflex, to boost your immune system and ease any pain.

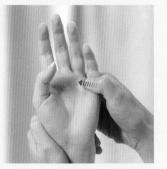

2 Next, work the ear reflex to improve circulation and remove toxins in the area. Finally, relax the body by working the solar plexus reflex.

Working the feet. This 5-minute routine can be done 3–4 times a week.

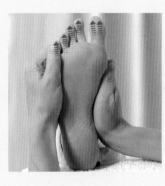

1 Begin with a few foot relaxation techniques. Then, starting at the bottom of the big toe, CW up each one of the toes until you reach the little toe. This will help clear congestion from the sinuses and release tension in your head.

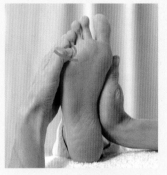

2 Work the ear reflex to improve circulation and to remove toxins in the area.

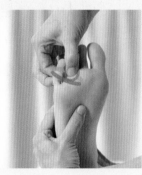

3 To work the inner ear reflex, place the tips of your right thumb and your right index finger between the second and third toes. Pinch gently several times. Work the solar plexus reflex to relax the body.

treating
travel sickness

Children especially can start feeling ill when traveling in a car, or on a bus or plane. When this occurs, ensure that there is adequate ventilation and make sure they stop reading and just relax. The following hand routine is designed to calm the body and help reduce nausea or anxiety.

This simple technique can help travel sickness subside quickly. For ease, it is best carried out on the hands.

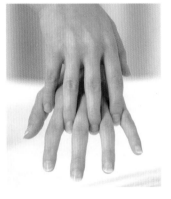

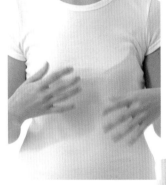

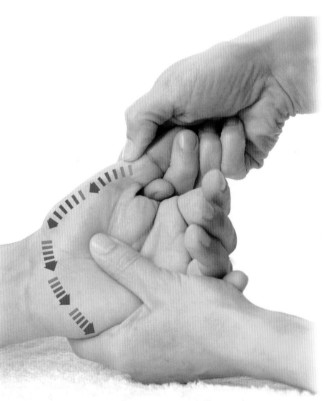

1 Begin with a few hand relaxation techniques, such as stroking, shown here.

2 Shaking both hands, keeping wrists loose, will help to expel negative energy and release tension.

3 Calm the nerves by working down the spine reflex.

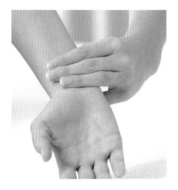

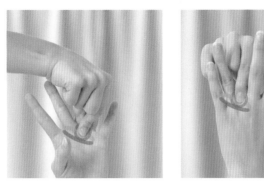

4 To help ease nausea, exert pressure with your index finger on the point on the forearm between the two wrist tendons. To find this exact spot, place three fingers across the wrist, with the ring finger touching the wrist crease and the index finger going up the arm. Keeping the tip of the index finger in place, the other fingers can then be lifted off.

6 Apply pressure to the eustachian tube reflex. Find this point by placing the tip of your right thumb and that of your right index finger between the second and third fingers on both the front and back of the hands. Pinch gently several times.

7 Finish by massaging the solar plexus reflex in both hands to calm the body.

5 Massage this point until the nausea disappears or is reduced. Massage the same point on the opposite forearm.

treating
babies and children

84

Babies enjoy being caressed, and evidence shows that it is beneficial for a baby's development to be touched and stroked. Because a baby's body is more sensitive to both touch and energy, only a few minutes of gentle, smooth pressure is needed to help reduce a range of complaints, from colic and constipation to diarrhea and irritability. This powerful way of communicating can also help mothers with postnatal "blues"—a few minutes of reflexology a day for mother and baby will help both to cope better.

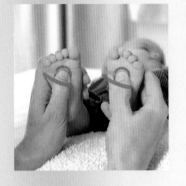

1 To help calm the baby, make eye contact and smile, gently rubbing the solar plexus reflex on both feet.

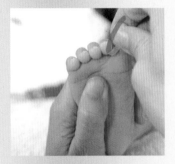
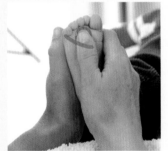

2 Starting with the big toe, gently rotate then squeeze each of the five toes on both feet. Gently massage the ball of each foot in a circular motion, starting on the inside of each foot and ending on the outside edge. This should ease any colic.

3 Starting on the outside edge of the right foot and using your thumb, make a gentle, smooth, circular motion over the digestive reflexes, in a clockwise direction. Repeat with the left foot, but start on the inside edge of the foot and end at the lower inside edge, just above the heel of the foot. This will help your baby with constipation or diarrhea.

Children

Children of all ages enjoy a few minutes of reflexology. They appreciate the attention and respond well to the treatment. However, make sure you keep the treatment short and fun, or the child might become restless.

A child's growing body goes through a bewildering number of changes in what can seem a short stretch of time. Whether a toddler or a teenager, reflexology can smooth the flow of energy in the various organs, and can help the child cope, both physically and emotionally, with this constant flux.

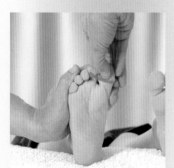 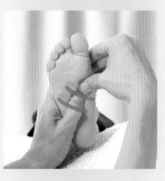 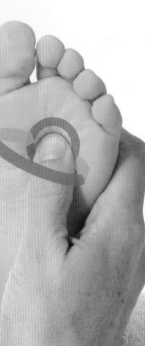

1 Begin with foot relaxation techniques—metatarsal kneading, toe rotation, thumb rolling, and foot wobbling are a good start. If the child is nine years of age or older, treat each one of the toes. Starting with the big toe, CW up the back of the toe once or twice, depending on the toe's size, working the whole area. Then, with your index finger, CW down the front of each of the toes. To help balance the hormones, gently squeeze the pituitary reflex, found on the fleshy part of the big toes, for a couple of seconds.

2 Release tension and relax the body by working down the spine reflex, starting just below the nail bed on the big toe and ending at the heel. Now work the shoulder reflex—it is surprising how many children, even at a young age, have tension in this area.

3 Gently massage the kidney and adrenal gland reflexes, then work the digestive system. Hold the uterus/prostate and ovary/testes reflexes, and stimulate them by rotating the foot with the other hand.

4 Using both hands, gently rub each foot's solar plexus reflex at the same time—this will help the child let go of certain emotions that they might be carrying.

self-help:
energy and vitality

We all go through periods in our life when our energy is more sluggish and our immune system is not as strong as it could be. We may feel depressed or emotional, lacking that extra "get up and go" to do the things we would like.

This 10-minute routine for the hands can stimulate your body's energy system, rebalancing your emotional and physical energies so that you feel uplifted. It can easily be practiced any time, or anywhere, whenever you feel the need to give yourself that extra boost.

3 First work the lung reflex, using the CW in all directions, then work across the diaphragm reflex in both directions. This will allow you to breathe in deeper, and make you feel "lighter" and more at ease.

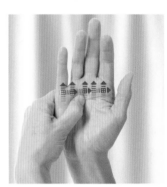

4 To relax your entire body, work down the spine reflex, starting just below the thumbnail and ending on the little finger side of the wrist crease. This will help to both stimulate and calm your nerves.

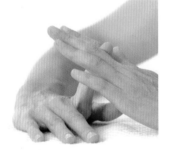

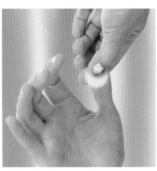

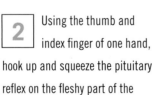

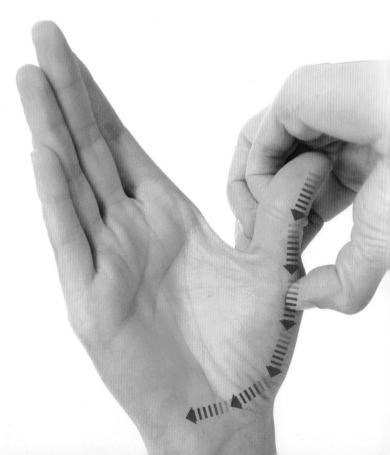

1 Warm up your hands for a few minutes with a few relaxation techniques, such as the finger stretch, shown here.

2 Using the thumb and index finger of one hand, hook up and squeeze the pituitary reflex on the fleshy part of the other hand's thumb, then change hands. This exercise will help to balance hormones.

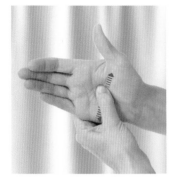 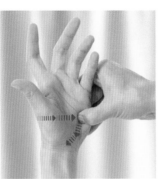 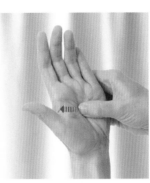 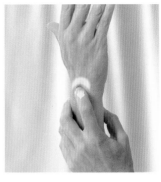

5 Work the large intestine reflex in both hands. Starting on the right palm at the ileo-caecal valve reflex, go up the ascending colon reflex, doing a right angle just below the waistline reflex. CW the transverse colon reflex, crossing the palm of the hand, extending to the left palm, and crossing all five zones. At the spleen reflex, between zones 4 and 5, turn another right angle, going down into the descending colon reflex. A short distance above the wrist, make another right angle turn into the sigmoid reflex, which extends across the palm above the wrist and ends in the rectum reflex, under the middle finger, by the bladder reflex.

6 With your thumb, CW over the pancreas reflex, found under the stomach reflex on the left hand. This will not only help balance your sugar levels, but will help you to spend less time worrying.

7 With your thumb, gently hook up into the natural dip found just above the wrist under the ring finger on the dorsal side of both hands. This is the sacro-ileac joint, and working this area will help release tension in your lower back.

8 Stimulate the adrenal glands and balance your energies by doing small circular movements over this reflex.

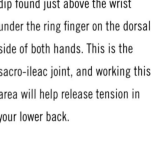

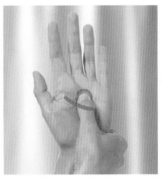

9 Finally, use your thumb to gently massage the solar plexus reflex on both hands. This will help balance your emotions, allowing you to let go of pent-up stress and negative thoughts.

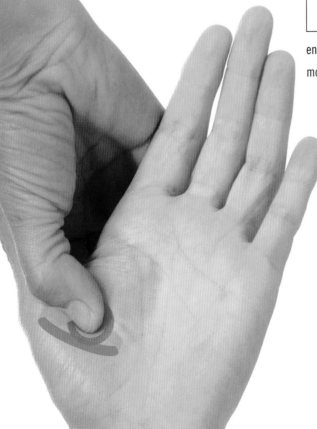

self-help:
relaxation

Working too hard, or having too much fun and insufficient rest or exercise, can quickly make us restless, nervous, or tense. Our surrounding environment can also make a difference. A crying baby, or a loud noise, for example, can easily make us feel "on edge."

This 20-minute routine, which can be done up to three times a week, will gently float these stresses and tensions away, not only relaxing and balancing our emotions but improving our physical well-being.

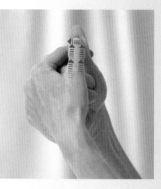

1 Warm up for a few minutes with some relaxation techniques, such as thumb and finger rotation. Then, with your thumb, hook up and squeeze the pituitary reflex on the fleshy part of both thumbs to help balance your hormones.

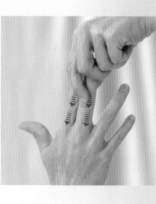

2 Repeat for the other fingers, but this time CW down the front of the fingers.

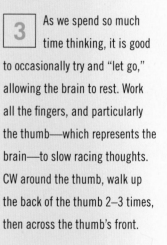

3 As we spend so much time thinking, it is good to occasionally try and "let go," allowing the brain to rest. Work all the fingers, and particularly the thumb—which represents the brain—to slow racing thoughts. CW around the thumb, walk up the back of the thumb 2–3 times, then across the thumb's front.

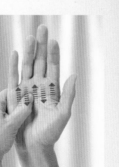

4 Work the lung reflex using the CW in all directions. This will help ease any tightness in the lungs and create a "lighter" feeling.

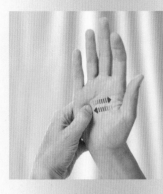
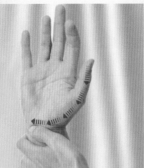
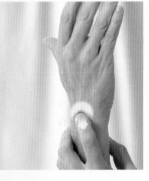

5 Work the diaphragm reflex in both horizontal directions. This will help you to relax and take deeper, more calming breaths.

6 To relax your entire body, work down the spine reflex, starting below the thumbnail and ending on the little finger side of the wrist crease. This will also help calm your nerves.

7 To "smooth," or even out, your internal energy and improve blood circulation, work the liver reflex on the right hand in a crisscross manner.

8 Now, hook up into the gallbladder reflex for a few seconds to aid digestion and help release tension in this area.

9 On the dorsal side of both hands, in the natural dip found above the wrist under the ring finger, work the sacro-ileac joint, gently hooking up using your finger. This will help release tension in the lower back. Finally, to help balance your emotions and "let go," use your thumb to gently massage the solar plexus reflex on both hands.

90

self-help:
metabolism
kickstart

Metabolic rates vary from person to person, and will change during different stages in a person's life. Reflexology can help balance this rate, bring us back into harmony with our bodies and minds, and make us feel more content and full of energy.

This routine, which should take about 15 minutes, can be carried out 2–3 times a week, and will provide a quick "boost."

1 Warm up for a few minutes with hand relaxation techniques, such as hand chopping, shown here.

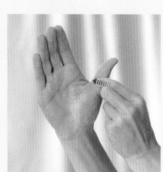

2 Use your thumb to hook up and squeeze the pituitary reflex on the fleshy part of both thumbs. This will balance your hormones and help you "get in touch" with your emotions.

3 Balance metabolism by stimulating your thyroid gland, found in the neck reflex on the palm side of both thumbs, on the "neck" part of the thumb. CW over this whole area.

4 Use the CW, in all directions, to work the lung reflex, then move across the diaphragm reflex, working in both directions. This will help you breathe more deeply.

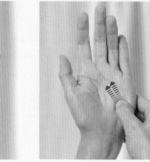

5 CW the stomach and spleen reflexes on the left hand, then move to the stomach reflex on the right hand. These reflexes are located between the diaphragm and waistline.

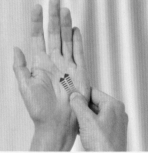

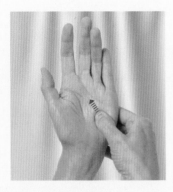
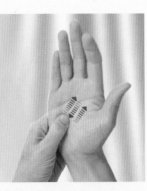
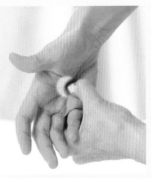
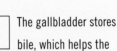
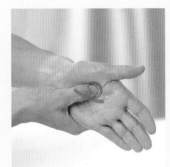

6 Working the stomach reflex on the left hand will stimulate your gastric juices and help digestion as well as automatically work the pancreas reflex that is situated under the stomach. The pancreas helps with maintaining the correct level of sugars in your bloodstream.

7 To help remove toxins from the bloodstream and improve blood flow, work the liver reflex. This is found on the right hand between the diaphragm and waistline, filling up most of this area and zones 3 to 5. CW this reflex in a crisscross manner with your thumb.

8 The gallbladder stores bile, which helps the body digest fatty substances. Work this reflex—found in zone 4, roughly in the middle of the liver reflex—by hooking it up with your thumb.

9 Help eliminate waste products from your body and regulate your water by working the kidney reflex. This bean-shaped reflex is found on both palms under the index finger, about one-third of the way up from the wrist crease. CW upward from this reflex, toward your thumb, then work the adrenal gland reflex by forming small circles slightly higher and to the thumb side of the kidney reflex.

10 Work the large and small intestine reflexes to help eliminate waste and toxins from your body, and to remove that bloating feeling. To help balance your emotions, and "let go," use your thumb to gently massage the solar plexus reflex on both hands.

self-help:
detoxification

It is easy for toxins to build up. Diet, stress, too much coffee, tea, or alcohol, and not doing sufficient exercise can all contribute. Environmental toxins, such as car fumes, can also increase toxin levels in our bloodstream.

Although there is plenty of literature on detox diets, this is outside the scope of this book. However, reflexology will help you to detoxify by improving circulation, eliminating toxins, promoting that feel-good factor, and bringing you back into harmony. Spend about 20 minutes twice a week doing this hand reflexology routine and notice the difference.

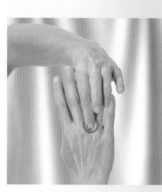

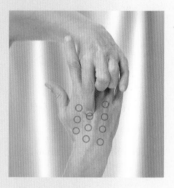

3 Massage the breast lymphatic system reflexes by pinching the web between each finger, starting at the thumb and ending with the little finger.

4 To improve immunity in your chest area, do a series of pinches to about halfway down the fleshy part of the palm; squeeze, returning up the hand.

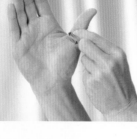

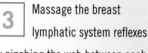

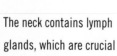

5 CW over the spleen reflex, on the left hand between the diaphragm line and waistline in zones 4 and 5. Working this reflex will help produce antibodies to fight infections.

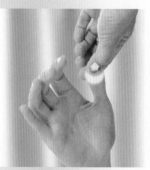

1 Warm up for just a few minutes with relaxation techniques. Using your thumb, hook up and squeeze the pituitary reflex on the fleshy part of both thumbs to balance your hormones.

2 The neck contains lymph glands, which are crucial to fighting infection and removing toxins. To stimulate these glands, CW the entire palm side of each "neck" area of your thumb.

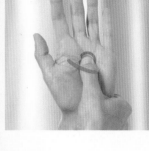
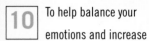

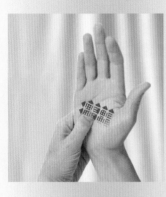

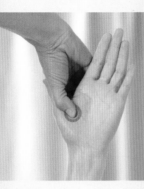

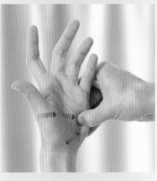

6 Remove toxins from the bloodstream and improve blood flow by working the liver reflex on the right hand between the diaphragm and waistline. CW this reflex in a crisscross manner with your thumb.

8 Work the adrenal gland reflex by forming small circles slightly higher and to the thumb side of the kidney reflex. Adrenal glands produce anti-inflammatory hormones that help produce that "feel-good" factor.

9 To help eliminate waste and toxins from your body, and to help get rid of that bloated feeling, work the large and small intestine reflex.

10 To help balance your emotions and increase a feeling of well-being, use your thumb to gently massage the solar plexus reflex on both hands.

7 Eliminate waste products from your body and regulate your water by working the bean-shaped kidney reflex (as shown here), found in both palms under the index finger, about one-third of the way up the palm from the wrist crease.

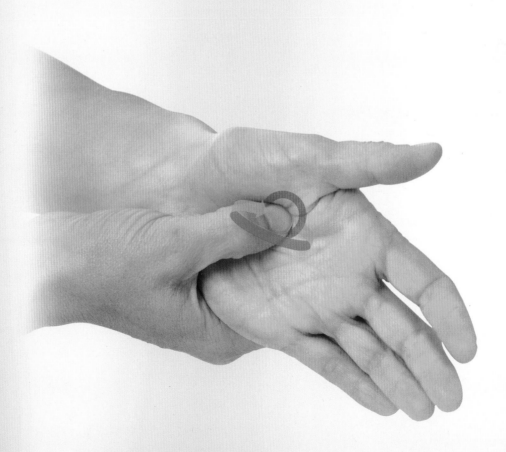

glossary

Abdominal area

The area of the body that starts at the diaphragm and extends under the lungs to the genitals.

Adrenal gland

A two-part gland situated just above each kidney. It is involved in the secretion of adrenalin, which increases the heart rate in response to stress.

Cardiovascular

Concerning the heart and/or the vast and intricate system of blood vessels that carry blood through the body.

Congestion

In reflexology, this means an area of the body where there is not a free flow of energy.

Diaphragm

The layer of muscles and tendons that separates the abdominal cavity from the chest cavity.

Eustachian tube

The canal from the middle ear to the back of the throat.

Holistic

Taken from the Greek word *holas,* which means "whole." In reflexology, it means that the person is treated as a whole, on a physical, mental, and spiritual level.

Hypothalamus

Part of the brain, containing a number of centers that control functions of the body, such as hunger, thirst, and temperature.

Meridians

The channels through which vital energy flows in the body, running to and from the hands and feet to the body and head.

Organ

A multicellular part of an animal, which forms a structural unit (such as the liver).

Reflex

An area found on the feet and hands that corresponds to a gland, an organ, or a part of the body.

Thoracic area

The area containing the heart and lungs. It is clearly marked off from the abdomen by the diaphragm.

Toxins

Substances that are poisonous to the body, which may be ingested in the food we eat or drink, or by other means.

Triple burner

Although there is no anatomical organ that correlates with the triple burner, the Chinese believe that all of the organs of the body are guarded by it.

Ureter

The duct that conveys urine from the kidney to the bladder.

Vital force

The life force or vital energy within us. The Chinese term is *Qi,* or *chi.*

Waistline

An imaginary line running horizontally across the foot and hand. On the foot it runs from the cuboid notch across to the other side of the foot.

Zone

In reflexology, any one of ten longitudinal sections through the body. Each contains one finger (or thumb) and one toe.

useful addresses

The Reflexology Association of America

4012 South Rainbow Bvd

P.O. Box 585

Las Vegas, NV 89 1032059

www.reflexology-usa.org

International Institute of Reflexology Inc.

5650 First Avenue North

P.O. Box 12642

St Petersburg, FL 33733-2642

email: iir@reflexology-usa.net

www.reflexology-usa.net

International Council of Reflexologists

PO Box 78060, Westcliffe Postal Outlet

Hamilton, ON L9C 7N5

Canada

email: icr@mountaincable.net

www.icr-reflexology.org

Associated Reflexologists of Colorado

P.O. Box 697 Englewood

Colorado 80151

www.reflexology-colorado.org

Georgia Reflexology Organization

P.O. Box 28031

Atlanta, GA 30358-8031

www.georgiareflexology.org

Reflexology Association of Illinois

P.O. Box 5515

Buffalo Grove, IL 60089-5515

www.reflexillinois.org

Maine Council of Reflexologists

P.O. Box 5583

Augusta

Maine 04330-5833

email: info@mcronline.org

www.reflexologyofmaine.org

Massachusetts Association of Reflexology

P.O. Box 80045

Stoneham, MA 01880

email: massreflexology@gmail.com

www.massreflexology.org

Reflexology Association of New Jersey

155 Franklin Avenue

Long Branch, NJ 07740

732-870-6831

www.njreflexology.org

New York State Reflexology Association

P.O. Box 262

Scarsdale, NY 10583

email: info@nysraweb.org

www.newyorkstatereflexology.org

North Carolina Reflexology Association

P.O. Box 480807

Charlotte, NC 28269

www.reflexology-nc.org

Reflexology Association of Ohio

1933 East Dublin-Granville Road,

136 Columbus, OH 43229

email: webmaster@reflexology-ohio.org

www.reflexology-ohio.org

Pennsylvania Reflexology Association

P.O. Box 215

Hershey, PA 17033

email: info@reflexologypa.org

www.reflexologypa.org

Washington Reflexology Association

P.O. Box 82857

Kenmore, WA 98028

email: info@washingtonreflexology.org

www.washingtonreflexology.org

Reflexology Organization of Wisconsin

904 Gail Place

Fort Atkinson, WI 53538

email: info@bexq.com

www.reflexologywi.org

index

Acknowledgements
Special thanks go to Joëlle Peeters for help with the photography. The publishers would also like to thank the following for the use of copyright material (bl = bottom left, l = left, bg = background):

Bridgeman Art Library: 7 (bl)
Corbis: cover images, 8, 11, 13 (bl), 20, 37
Getty: 22, 64
istock photography: 9 (bg), 35
Photos.com: 12, 15, 21, 65
Topfoto: 6 (l)